THE NO B.S. GUIDE TO SUSTAINABLE W8 LOSS

THE NO B.S. GUIDE TO SUSTAINABLE W8 LOSS

8 SIMPLE STEPS TO TROUBLESHOOTING YOUR WEIGHT LOSS

JOHN GAGLIONE

Cover Design: Tri Widyatmaka
Interior Design: Daniel Ojedokun

Disclaimer

This book is designed to provide information and motivation to the reader. It is provided with the understanding that the author and/or publisher is not engaged to render any type of psychological, legal, or any other kind of professional advice. The content found within is the sole expression and opinion of its author.

No warranties or guarantees are expressed or implied by the author's and/or publisher's choice to include any of the content in this volume. Neither the publisher nor the author shall be liable for any physical, psychological, emotional, financial, or commercial damages, including, but not limited to special, incidental, consequential or other damages.

1st edition, July 2021

Printed in the United States of America

Table of Contents

Introduction

Cue The DJ Khaled Saying...

Another One!

That's probably what you're thinking about when you see yet another book about weight loss. Another book that is about to prescribe to you the all-in-one solution to solving every single weight loss problem you've ever had. *THIS* diet is going to be the best thing since the word *DIET* was invented or *THIS* workout program will have you in your best summer body in just a few weeks. You'll see words like *"FAST, QUICK, SHORTCUTS"* plastered all over with your most troubling or most desirable body part on the other side of that phrase.

Does this seem at all familiar?

It should because, quite frankly, the health and fitness market is a big one. The reality is that because so many people have a desire to be healthy and to get fit, the new inventions, the new diets, and the new workouts are not going anywhere. Now, please do not take this as my public declaration that all of this is bad. This is not my position with regards to the health and fitness industry. What this communicates to me is the desire many people have to be healthy and fit, which I feel is an incredible thing. In fact, count me as one of them! I personally care about my health and fitness. I care about my body and understand how it plays a role in how I see myself, how I see the world, and everything else that comes along the ride called life.

So you might be asking the question— if I know that the health and fitness category is saturated with the new blues, then why would I consider joining the merry-go-round and take the time to write a book myself?

Let me tell you why.

This book was born out of a need. I've always found that my own nutrition and my own body weight have been areas I've struggled with throughout my childhood and throughout my adult life. If you look at the news and see stories and statistics about health, fitness, and weight-loss, it's obvious that I am not alone in this. Just looking at the United States, we can see that obesity, diabetes, and heart diseases are continuing to rise, leading to all sorts of other health problems, mental health issues, and so much more.

With so much information available on dieting, nutrition, weight loss, and exercise, you would think that these issues would be trending downward, not upward, but that is not the case. The information alone has not resulted in changes, or at least not in change that is sustainable.

Also, considering the times we are in as I write, has our health ever been more important than it is today? Our health impacts all the areas of our lives. It's not just a question of how we appear in front of a mirror. How is our confidence and our mental health impacted when we do not have a handle on our physical health? The pandemic brought this to light for many of us. No longer was health and fitness a luxury, but a priority that we need to have. It makes the phrase "health is wealth" more real when factors bring to light what quality of life we have when our health is not in gear. This is a component that many health and fitness books cover on the surface, at best, to fit their own objectives rather than diving into the depth of its true impact on our overall lives.

Reflecting on this situation made me look at my own weight loss journey and realize that something is missing or just not quite right. Why do people like me, who have the desire to maintain a healthy lifestyle, find it so hard to do so EVEN with so much information out there on how to do EXACTLY that. It's here that the genesis of this book occurred and it is now a tangible thing you're holding in your hand.

I wrote this book to hopefully help people like us, those who want to lose weight, to be able to know the difference between tried and true weight loss principles versus "here today, gone tomorrow" tactics. These tactics do just that with our weight loss results. They are here today and gone tomorrow. Being sick and tired of this reality, I wanted to figure it out. Is there a way to lose weight and maintain that weight loss. Is there a way to get the scale needle to move in the direction I want, when I want, and be able to keep it there without questioning if the scale is broken, or wrong, or conjuring up some other reasoning to make me feel just a little bit better about myself?

I can remember a time when one of my mentors shared a line that really helped to put things in perspective. He said, "if information is all that was required to change lives, then all the lives would have been changed by now".

At first, I did not fully comprehend what he meant, but boy do I understand it now. There is a wealth of knowledge available, more than we would ever need to know about, on how to move the needle on the scale and also keep that needle in the desired direction we want. I wondered, what if someone could go ahead and cut through a lot of the B.S. that is out there?

What if someone who has gone through many diets like the ones listed below could extract the commonalities of all of them and put it into one easy to follow and easy to adjust approach?

SOME of The Diets I've Done (I'm sure you know about 10-15 more that can go on this list):

- The Low Carb Diet
- The Keto Diet
- The Macro Counting Diet
- The Calorie Cycling Diet
- The Carb Cycling Diet

As someone who has done all these diets without ever seeing any sustainable changes, I realized that something is up. Something is just not quite right. What I uncovered was that these diets very rarely ever address making lifestyle habits. When following these diets, I've lost some weight only to see that weight come back on like an ex that you were trying to keep in the past!

Over time I've seen and been part of the 21-day challenges or the 6 weeks to [insert goal here]. All good ideas, but because they were designed for a period of time, that is how long my results lasted… for a period of time. This is where the big epiphany hit me like a ton of bricks. We really don't have a weight loss problem. What we have is a weight maintenance problem. People lose weight all the time. What people aren't able to do is to keep the weight off! It's this problem that the book in your hand will tackle and address. Now, before I move forward, let me tell you what this book does not tackle. It does not tackle how to maintain weight quickly. It's not a quick fix. It's not some magic pill or silver dollar or lucky charms kind of book. It's real information about what actually makes maintained weight loss possible. The contents will show you how to produce sustainable results over time and not just stop at a period of time like 6 weeks or 12 weeks. We will cut through the noise of the gimmicks and fads out there in the fitness industry and identify the elements that make a difference in the long run.

Worth Noting…

What's in this book is not coming from someone who has no experience in the fitness industry. Not only have I tried the diets and various weight loss programs, but I've also served hundreds, if not thousands, as a strength coach for over 14 years. Over almost 2 decades of being in this space, what has frustrated me the most is not being able to walk the talk of having a healthy, sustainable lifestyle. Yes, I found tremendous success in powerlifting and helped many others do the same, but when it came to having a handle on my own weight, my own level of fitness, and my own nutrition, those results were nowhere to be found.

One Size Doesn't Fit All Perfectly

Speaking of unfounded results, I believe one of the reasons why many have a challenging time handling their own weight, level of fitness, or nutrition is that the solutions typically presented in the health and fitness industry are not shared in a way that is suitable or sustainable for people.

Typically the solutions are presented in a one size fit all model. They do not take into consideration the many different factors that can impact one's response to a generalized approach. Too often the information is generalized without any form of customization or education for the consumer to be able to answer the question: how can I tweak this for ME, so that I can use what works and throw away what doesn't?

It's a lot sexier or a lot easier to say, "do this ONE diet, or ONE program, and your weight loss dreams will come true". It's a lot harder to say, "here's this one diet and the things to consider depending on who you are and how you can make that diet or program work for you".

In thinking about this further, I began to question what is in this book and who the information BEST serves. I'll admit this is a tough question to answer because the information in this book, in all honesty, can help anyone no matter where they are in their fitness journey. However, the imperative word in the question is BEST. In evaluating my own journey and the successes and struggles along the way, I discovered who this book can best serve and who it's not best for. I'll address the latter first.

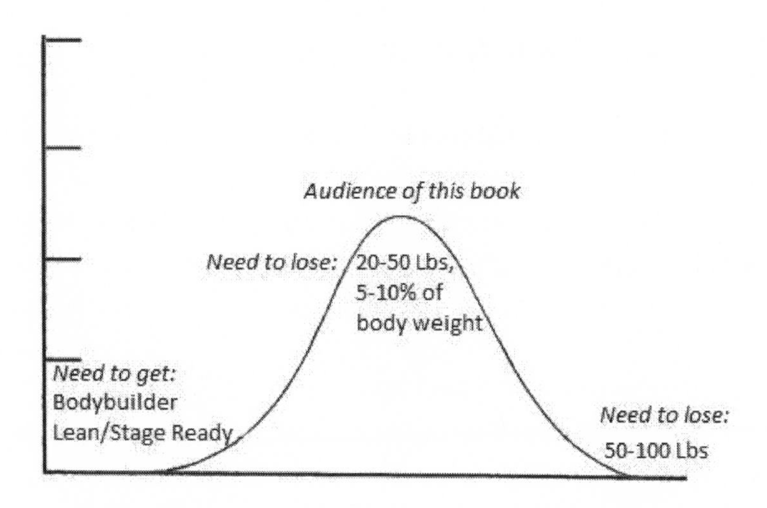

This book is not best for someone who finds themselves in the extreme part of their weight loss journey. Imagine a bell curve as shown in the image below.

If you find yourself at the edges, whether you're looking to get super lean like you were about to compete at a bodybuilding show or you find yourself needing to lose north of 50 pounds, maybe 100 pounds or more, this book is not BEST for you. This does not mean there isn't information, as I shared earlier, that can be beneficial, but is it BEST? No. What is best for those who find themselves in those areas? Enlisting the assistance of a coach. In those situations, typically, the journey is longer and it requires far more specification and precision than one could address within the scope of a book like this. You'll learn later that before I was able to enter the shaded ideal target range of weight loss, I found myself at the far right end and needed to enlist the services of a coach to get me to where I needed to be, where I could empower my own weight loss journey.

The ideal audience for this book are those who find

themselves needing to lose 20-50 pounds, or about 5-10% of their current body weight. It's this group of people that I ideally wrote this book for, as they could take the checklist that we will be sharing later and be empowered to make the necessary changes in their habits to create the health and fitness results they want and to keep them. If you've tried a bunch of diets, programs, or maybe have even yo-yoed in your health and fitness journey, you're about to get the tools to manipulate your body weight up or down depending on your goals. By the end of this book, you'll know the framework to work in and know how to troubleshoot any areas that are lagging to help you accomplish the goals you want time and time again.

Troubleshooting

This is the first "Troubleshooting" section of the book. Everyone has a different situation, a different biology, and different goals, so everyone needs an individual approach. The goal of this book is to help you craft that approach yourself and stick to it. These sections will prompt you to respond to the points made in the book, allowing you to tailor the advice to your needs, find the trouble spots in your lifestyle and habits, and begin to construct a program that works for you. Let's get started!

- What diets or fitness routines have you tried in the past? What things were successful about the diet? What was unsuccessful? What did you learn from it or struggle with? For example, perhaps you tried a ketogenic diet and curbed your hunger, but experienced a brain fog and poor performance at the gym, or felt overly restricted. Write out your answers below!

- Were you able to sustain any long-term habits from those diets? What are those habits? Which habits did you fall off with when stopping the diet?

- Where are you on your weight-loss journey? How much time have you spent trying to lose weight? How many pounds do you need to lose to hit your goal? Where are you on our bell curve above?

- What is unique about your situation coming into this journey? For example, you may be a busy mom, have food allergies, or be coping with an injury. Note anything that would add a layer of difficulty or specificity to your program or potentially create the need for a more customized approach.

WHAT MAKES THIS BOOK DIFFERENT THAN OTHER HEALTH/WEIGHT LOSS BOOKS...

It's the framework and the education provided to help you troubleshoot your own way to your weight loss goals that makes this book both exciting and different. It's not built on becoming America's next diet or to be tomorrow's newest infomercial. It's informational, practical, repeatable, foundational, and, most importantly, effective. You will uncover the areas in your health and fitness that need to be tweaked so that you hit the mark with your goals every time. For example, fixing my sleep was my trouble area. My inability to see consistent and sustainable success within my weight loss journey was not because I did not train or have a diet to follow. As a powerlifter, there was a ton of effort and focus in my training. Through the checklist featured in this book, I was able to uncover the fact that my recovery and stress management was really way off. These are topics that typically aren't addressed when it comes to weight loss. Once I got my sleep under control, that is when things began to change for me. How beneficial would it be for you to know where those sticking points are for you? How powerful and liberating would it be to know how to move past those sticking points and see your weight loss goals move in the right direction?

A big part of finding success in this journey is knowing what buttons to press. This is different for everyone and, until the tools that I share with you in this book were put in a simplified way to follow, the success part escaped me. I'm glad that won't be the case for you. No more wasted efforts in areas that aren't causing you issues. No more diet hopping thinking that the next diet is "the one". Remember there is no one size fits all perfectly, but we can uncover what is getting in the way of you getting there and empower you with tools, strategies, and a framework to ensure you get there. Are you excited yet?

The What and Where Of The Troubleshooting Guide to W8 Loss

At my heaviest, at the beginning of this journey, I was 340 pounds with over 40% body fat.

Fast-forward to today and I can say that at my lowest in this journey I was able to weigh 198 pounds and have been able to keep at least 100 pounds off consistently since then. This was not an overnight process, however. This is a 5-year journey of mine. You might be thinking right now, "I don't have 5 years to lose this weight, I want it now". I know that feeling all too well. I've also learned that how fast I lost weight also determined the speed at which it came back.

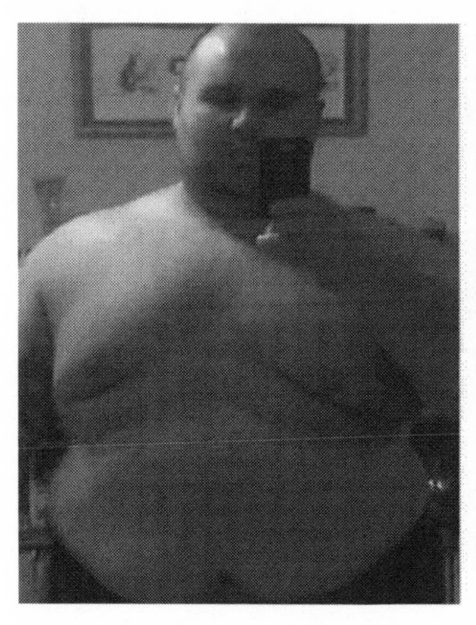

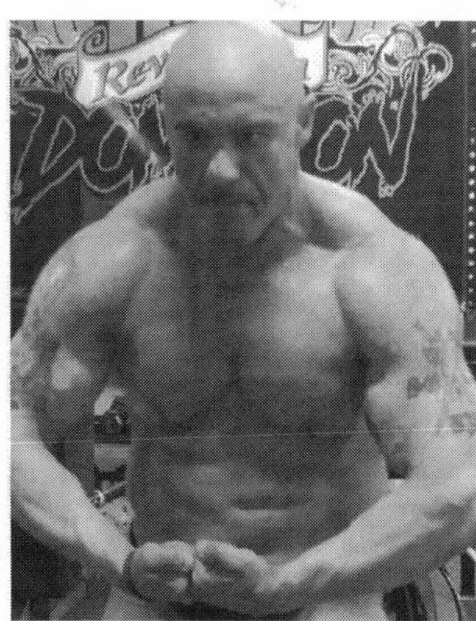

There's a quote by Steve Jobs where he says, "you never can connect the dots going forward but you can looking back". That is what happened to me when it came to this troubleshooting guide. Going forward. I did not see how the components of this book worked. The overwhelming amount of information out there made it very easy to overlook what it really takes to get results. Looking back though I can see what really moved the needle for me. I discovered what really created the kind of results that I can sustain over a long period of time. When you go through this book, keep in mind that slow and steady will win you the race and the races to come thereafter. I hope I have not lost you yet. We are almost ready to jump into the checklist and start showing you how you can begin to put this into practice starting today. Before I break down the journey we are about to embark on, however, I feel that it is important that you truly understand the depth of where I'm writing from. I would venture a guess that you too have a similar journey or path in your life.

CHAPTER 1

THE BACKSTORY...(WHERE IT ALL BEGAN)

My entire life.

That's how long the struggle with weight has been for me.

How long has your struggle been?

From the earliest that I can remember, I was chubby. In elementary school, I could not play football because I could never make the weight class. I was the big kid growing up. This identity haunted me for a big part of my life. Body image issues would come soon after.

Then came high school where I began wrestling. It was there I found some success. I went from 275 pounds all the way down to 189 pounds, eventually settling in at the 215 weight class my senior year. I then started competing in powerlifting as a teenager in the 198 class. That was great for me. I once again found some success. I found something that I was good at and it was working for me.

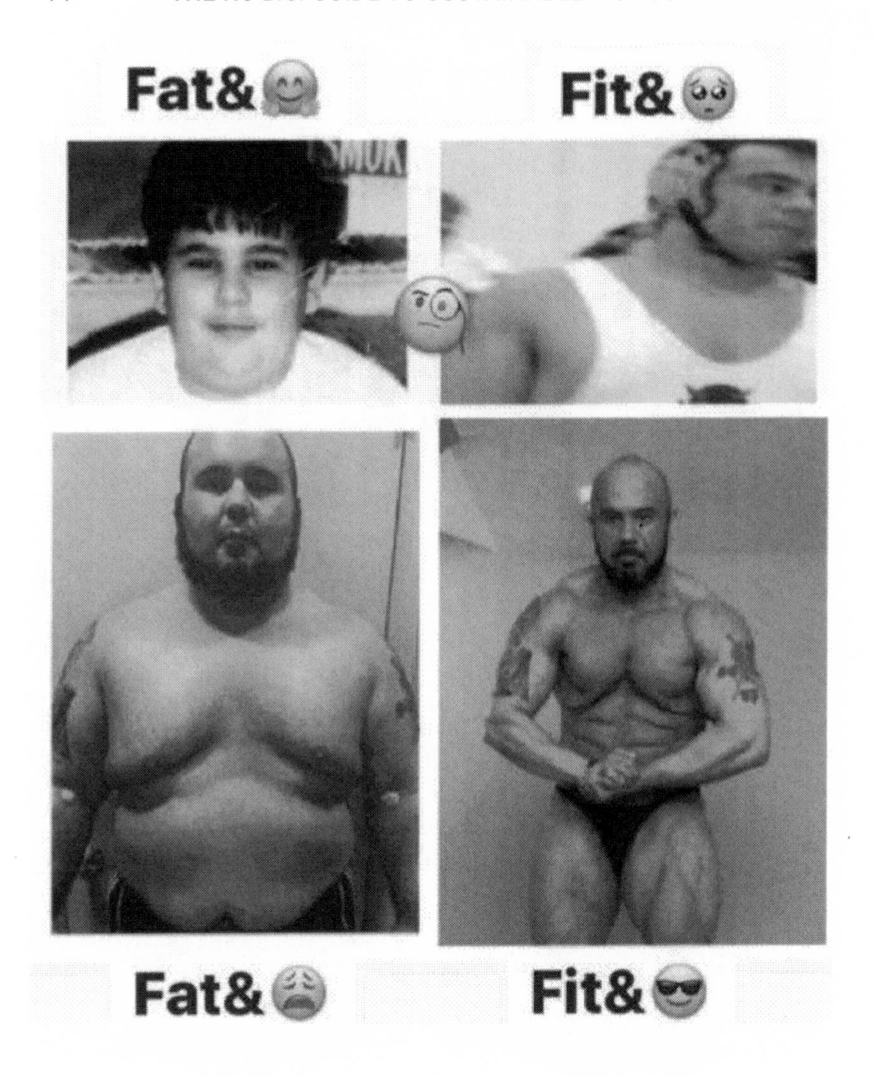

Strength Becoming A Weakness

You've gone too far.

Have you ever heard this said before? When you are doing the right thing or something is working, but then it gets out of hand? Well, that is what happened to me. You see, I found success with powerlifting and it was working for me, but what also happened was my activity level dropped because I stopped wrestling. My new obsession became the barbell (powerlifting). Sure, it started off as a healthy hobby. Lifting weights is not bad and I loved it! The question that I now ask myself though, is "Did you love it too much?". The Harvard Business Review had an article on leadership where they shared that taking strengths too far can become a weakness. For example, take someone who is a do-it-all type of person. That is a strength, the ability to do everything. It becomes a weakness when you are trying to do things bigger or faster. It's at those times the strength gets exposed as a weakness as no one person can do everything well and fast. For me, my strength led me to squatting 900 pounds in competition as a powerlifter. That was a goal of mine which was a long time coming.

As I climbed the powerlifting ranks, so did my weight. My first meet was back in 2006 where I squatted 375 pounds. Over the years, I would climb to 400, 500, 600 and did my first 800-pound squat in 2013. When I hit the 800 pounds mark, things began to slow down for me. Yes, it was my first nationally ranked lift, but I also was 283 pounds at the time. I had come a long way from the days of the 198 class. I was almost 100 pounds heavier. Seeing that, I thought that it was time to lose this weight before it got out of control, but then came the other part of me. That part of me that was a powerlifter and that part of me thought, "wow I'm close to 900 pounds, why don't I push for that?". This would become my new obsession. I was willing to do anything to hit the 900 pounds mark, even at the expense of my health. This was a big deal for me.

10 years in the making...

I did it! 900 pounds! I had set my mind to hit this monumental moment and accomplished it, but the celebration was short. At the time, my grandfather was sick and did not have very much more life to live. My family and I got on a plane to South Carolina to see him. It was then that I saw my grandfather alive for the last time. He passed away shortly after. This was in 2016, 10 years after I started powerlifting.

That is when I started doing some reflection. Here I am with this 900 pound squat, but I don't feel great. I was not able to sleep well. I woke up in pain most mornings. I had trouble doing normal things, such as tying my shoes and, get this, I was afraid to play beach volleyball and do other kinds of activities for fear that I would tear a muscle. At this point, I was simply existing but not really living life. Then I thought about how I was a coach preaching health, preaching being strong both inside and outside of the gym, but was not living it. I preached a good game, but I was not living what I was preaching. I wasn't leading by example. I had to do something to turn things around.

Turning Tides

Tony Robbins, a famous motivational speaker/life coach, says that "it's in our decisions that our destiny is shaped". I had to make a few decisions of my own to ensure that my destiny was not going to end up negatively. The first decision I made was to go to Red Bank, New Jersey to a facility called The Nutrition Treatment Center run by Dr. Tom Bilella. There, I got my blood work done and my body fat done. The results? I was 335 pounds, had 40 plus percent body fat, bad vitamin levels, and an array of other health issues. It was all information that no one wants to hear, but it is what I NEEDED to know in order to turn the tide.

The next thing I did was to get a sleep study done. Remember how I shared that I would wake up in pain and never had a great night of sleep? I thought it would be important to find out why this was happening. That is where I found out that I had bad sleep apnea which prevented me from being able to recover well from my training. Knowing this information gave me power. It helped me to learn what I needed and why I felt as I did. With this clarity, I began to feel empowered. With this new found information, I was able to get better rest which allowed me to put more energy into my training and into my nutrition, along with everything else in my life.

Shifting Gears

Now came the time for me to drop weight. It was important to me that I do this for my health and to walk the talk as a coach. It's at this point some people might say that to drop what you were, you have to drop what got you there. Powerlifting got me there. Powerlifting contributed to me neglecting my activity levels that I had during wrestling, but it was also what I identified with the most. I identified as a powerlifter. So, there were two things I could do.

Option A: Continue focusing on Powerlifting

Option B: Focus on Weight Loss

I chose option C.

What's Option C, you ask? Use my love for powerlifting but pivot by approaching it differently. I decided to make a deal with myself to begin participating in competitions but at different weight classes.

In powerlifting you have super heavyweight, the 308 weight class, the 242 weight class, the 220 weight class, the 198 weight loss, and so on. I decided that I would have the goal of getting healthier, losing weight, and made it my new focus to go down one weight class at a time while still competing in the sport that I loved so much.

In 2018, I competed in my first meet after devising this strategy. I competed in the 242 weight class. Yep, that's right 242! The last time I was 242 pounds was in 2008! Another 10 year mark. Guess how much I squatted? 770 pounds! So close to 800 while being almost 100 pounds lighter than my heaviest weight. Being so close to 800 I decided to set a new goal for myself.

I'm going to squat 800 pounds in six weight classes!

Over the next two to three years I would use this as my north star. It allowed me to continue to have performance driven goals, to maintain a lot of muscle mass, and have some fun along the way too. The cool thing about this also was that it helped me to not be so consumed by the scale. It was important for me to lose the weight, but sometimes that battling of perfection can overwhelm you. I'm glad that was not the case for me.

For your journey, it is important that you identify the things you love to do and, before removing them altogether, find out how they can be done differently. I did not choose to stop powerlifting, I just decided to use it differently. The more fun you can make this journey, the more likely you will be able to stick to it. It's that part we hate about diets and programs. They are too static. They aren't easy going or easily adjustable. They are more concrete than clay. You can't reinvent them or configure new approaches with them.

Now you're probably wondering, did I get it done? Was I able to meet my goal of squatting 800 in six different weight classes? The answer...

Yes.

It took several years, but I was able to do it and the lightest I did it, after 14 years as a powerlifter, was in the 198 weight class. Over 140 pounds of weight loss. It's at that point I decided that I would take the next step.

Shifting Gears Again

I would do my first bodybuilding competition. Say what, Gagz? Bodybuilding competition?! I figured that if I can go from obese to stage ready lean that it would be an inspiration to many others of what's possible. Perhaps they would be able to see themselves overcome the struggle of losing 20-50 pounds. I wanted to not just talk about it being possible. I wanted to serve as a coach and show that it was possible by walking the talk.

So I decided to shift gears once again, a common theme you will see in this book. Because of what I know, I have the power to change courses and accomplish whatever I put my mind to. You'll be able to do the same.

Now I'll be honest and tell you that it wasn't easy. I do not want to make it out to seem like there is no effort and no frustration along this journey. That is not the case. In fact, when I was entering the bodybuilding competition, I was doing so during the pandemic, which made things a lot more challenging. I had over six cancellations for shows which turned my six-month diet into a 10-month diet. But I came too far to not finish what I started. I thought of you. I thought of how awesome it would be to be an example of what could be. So, I pushed through. I stayed committed to the goal I set my mind to at the beginning of this journey. I continuously saw my goal and let that guide me. Keep your eyes on the prize. That's how I got there. Stuff will happen, but you are bigger and better than those things.

Are you ready to create your own version of this story now...

I shared this extended version of my backstory because I wanted you to see that the road is not straight. There are detours, there are pit stops, there are frustrations, and there are plenty of imperfections, but there is a way to still arrive at the destination.

Now, many may say after reading this that, because I am a strength coach and had a background in lifting weights already, it was inevitable that I would find success. They may say that they cannot relate to what I did. But this is the very reason I went through the journey I did and mapped it out in this book. It's not just for someone who has an extensive background in training. What you're about to dive into isn't centered around your training expertise or the extensive background of your training. The book is designed to help anyone drop the weight they want and to get to a healthier lifestyle.

In fact, I've worked with several men and women who have lost 20 to 30 pounds. They were not strength coaches or elite powerlifters. They are regular men and women like you. My dad even decided to join in and he's lost 30 pounds and kept it off. And get this... he wasn't perfect along the journey and you don't have to be either.

These results show that when you know the principles that I'm about to share with you, you can get sustainable weight loss. These 8 steps on the checklist here will guide you on exactly how to tweak your health and fitness lifestyle to meet the goals that you have.

In this book you will get:

- The mindset you need to master your own weight loss journey.
- A detailed breakdown of what the checklist is and how to navigate it.
- The importance of recovery and why you don't want to ignore it if you want stellar, consistent results.
- The basics essentials of exercising (you don't need to become an elite powerlifter to get elite results)
- The basic essentials of nutrition that are simple to implement.

So, without further delay, let's just get into this journey. I cannot wait to see you at the end of the road. Remember that your goal is possible. You just have to see it first. Let's find your north star right now.

Troubleshooting Your Weight-Loss Journey

- What have been your 3 biggest obstacles with weight maintenance in your life?

____

____

- Highlight one or more major turning point in your awareness of the effects of your lifestyle? For example, getting my sleep apnea under control and improving my sleep quality was the catalyst for the start of my successful weight loss effort.

____

____

- What helps you stay on track and follow your plans to lose and maintain your weight more effectively? For example, one thing that helps curb my cravings is utilizing protein powder as a flavoring to make an otherwise unhealthy dessert healthier. Another example would be utilizing longer fasting periods or tighter feeding windows in order to create a larger calorie deficit, so that I can enjoy a bigger treat meal later on in the day or week while accounting for those calories.

____

____

CHAPTER 2

SEE YOUR GOAL

Throwback Moment.

Do you remember the days of MapQuest? For those who may not be familiar, it's a web-based platform used back in the day to get driving directions. This was before the times of GPS which we now have access to easily on our smartphone devices. All we have to do today is enter where we want to go and our app automatically tells us the directions to get to our destination. Like using a GPS when heading on a journey, we need to have the same tool for our weight loss journey in order for it to be successful. A GPS is only good when it's given a destination. The destination must be determined before the directions. As we embark on our weight loss journey, before we can identify the action steps necessary on the checklist, it's important to know the destination. What goal would you like to accomplish? The goal is our north star. It's the lamp that lights up the road and allows us to remain focused on the journey ahead.

Before beginning any journey establishing the destination is key. It's important that you determine what that destination is for you and not have someone else do it for you. Take a moment to think of that right now.

What goal would you like to accomplish? What goal do you have the motivation to work toward? What goal would make you happy to sustain? For me, it was getting back to my weight in high school while still being able to maintain my muscle mass and still feel strong. That was my aim. What's yours? Knowing where you are going is step one in the battle. Without knowing that, the remaining steps of our checklist won't have value for you. I want you to imagine the checklist as guardrails on the highway. It helps to keep you on the road so that you are able to reach your destination. The checklist is your navigation tool.

The checklist by itself, however, is not going to do the work. That is on you. Like a GPS when we enter a destination, we still have to do the driving. That will be no different for you in this journey, but you will know the directions. You will know how to get there and that, in and of itself, is an empowering feeling.

Types of Goals

When constructing your goals, as with navigating to your destinations, it's important to create two types of goals. This is where a lot of diets and fitness programs go wrong. They are designed typically for one of these types and not both. Most diet plans will tell you how to lose 25 pounds in 8 weeks. That is a great short term result, but what happens after the 8 weeks? Do I gain all the 25 pounds back? Do I gain some of it back? Can I extend this diet plan past 8 weeks? These are all legitimate questions that we need to ask, especially when we want to get off the merry-go-round of losing weight only to gain it all back and then some.

That is why I suggest having both short-term goals and long-term goals. This will allow you to be able to create results repeatedly and be able to have them stay for a longer period of time. As I write this to you, I'm able to still walk around well over 100 pounds lighter than when I was at my heaviest and that is because I consistently incorporate the concepts of both short and long term goals.

When it came to my goals, I knew I wanted to get back to being in the 198 pound weight class. Starting from 340 plus pounds though meant that this would be a little longer of a journey than that of someone who needed to lose just 20 pounds. Because of this, I set this as my long term goal. If you have a big goal that seems a bit unattainable from where you are today, do not be discouraged. Instead, set that as your long term goal. If you have 50 pounds to lose, let that be your long term goal. Remember this journey is not about perfection. It's about progression. It's about constantly improving day by day, week by week, and, before you know it, years later you will master your body and will be able to gain and lose weight intentionally rather than be helpless in the always-changing hands of the diet and fitness industry.

Once I established my long term goal, I developed short term goals to help me stay encouraged and keep me motivated along the way. Starting at 340 pounds, I made my first goal to get to 308 pounds. My short term goal was to drop 32 pounds, not drop 142 pounds. Do you see how much more doable dropping 32 pounds is compared to 142 pounds? For you, if you're starting out and want to drop 50 pounds, perhaps your short term goal would be 10 pounds, which is one fifth of that. If you want to go even smaller, you can go one tenth of that and start off dropping 5 pounds from the outset.

After hitting 308, I then transitioned to 275, and then to 242, and then to 220, and so on until I reached my last stop of 198. Because I was able to do this gradually, I was also able to learn a lot about the process of how to do it and keep it off as well. Another nugget that I got from this journey that I would like to share with you is that your short and long term goals do not have to be limited to just the pounds on the scale, although that is a big one for the purpose of this book. Because I was empowered by the checklist, I was able to shift back and forth through various goals. I was able to accomplish strength goals, aesthetic goals, and other health goals because of this process. Again, when you are aware of the process, you can have total control on how it goes. That's what excites me most about providing this information for you. You can get behind the wheel of your weight loss journey and drive the car to where you want to go.

Picking Weekly Goal Setting

I have two more things I want to share with you when it comes to goals before I fully lay out all the components of the checklist which I know you are eagerly waiting for and probably already skipped ahead to! But please do not skip this! It's important that the foundation is set in order to make the most of the system. This is all foundational work that is often skipped or overlooked and that prevents sustainable results. It is important to make sure that, when moving forward with your goal, that goal is something that you are able to see regularly. This means breaking it down even more to weekly goals. We started off with a zoomed out look at our goals, but we don't live zoomed out. We live day by day and week by week. Weekly goals allow us to be able to see where we are before we advance past the point where we are able to tweak our plan and make the necessary adjustments to keep the car moving along in our journey.

When setting weekly goals you want to look at Sunday through Saturday typically. The goal is to build our way towards having perfect weeks, which cannot happen without having perfect days. As you'll see in this book, one thing leads to another. We go from a big goal, then drill down to the week, and then drill down even further with the daily. Because this is not a copy and paste approach, you will have to utilize everything you've done through this process to instruct you on what your next steps should be.

What does that look like on a practical level, you ask? Review what your previous week looked like and see what areas of improvement that you can shift your focus to this week so that you are consistently making progress and moving forward towards your overall goal. For example, sometimes I might identify that an area of improvement is my sleep. Perhaps I'm not getting the sleep I need and thus it's impacting what my recovery looks like, which we will talk about later on. Because I know this information about this desired area of improvement, I can now shift that to be my weekly focus, along with addressing other relevant factors you'll see in the checklist.

The goal of the checklist is to be able to identify the actions we need to take on a regular basis. It's designed to address both the weekly and daily progress so that all bases are covered and you can ensure that you are working towards your long term goals with confidence and achieving success as you progress overall.

Assessing Wins

As we master individual days with the checklist, we will then be able to label those as wins. Assessing wins is the second thing I want to address. It's important that we are able to not just be aware of what we are doing, or even just be aware of the actions we need to take, but be able to track when we are doing those actions versus when we are not. Consider it like a scoreboard. If there was no scoreboard, how would we actually know the score? The score dictates what play we run on the court. Similarly, when we know what is working, when we have a winning streak because we are able to check off the 8 things on the checklist repeatedly, we can then turn those winning days into winning weeks which lead to us winning the challenge of sustainable weight loss.

In the next chapter, you're going to find out exactly what wins we should be aiming for, but just remember two things. First, you're going to need to track whether you won. Second, you must have a goal in mind that you are working towards, both in the short and long term realm. Let's get to the checklist!

Troubleshooting Your Goals

- If we could wave a magic wand over your weight-loss journey, what would you like to see happen? What changes do you want to see in your body composition and lifestyle?

- What would you be willing to sacrifice in order to achieve that result? What are your non-negotiables that you are not willing to sacrifice to achieve that result?

- Take a moment, imagine that you are looking in the mirror and have achieved your desired result. Write down how you would feel in that moment.

- Why is this feeling important to you? What does this feeling give you? Who or what else in your life may benefit from your transformation?

- Write down your primary smart goal. Put it somewhere visible so that you can see it every single day. Add words or images to remind you of why and for who or what you are pursuing this goal. This is your anchor.
- Write down some short term goals

- Write down some long term goals

____

____

- What are the daily and weekly actions which will lead to your goals? For example, consider any of the habits on our checklist in the next chapter or other actions you need to take to start incorporating those habits into your life. List 4-5 things you can do.

____

____

CHAPTER 3

CHECKLIST EXPLAINED

This is what you got this book for.

The checklist! If I were a betting man, I would bet that you sped right through the previous sections to see this section specifically. If you did, I strongly suggest that you go back to the introduction and read the section about goal setting. The foundation laid down in those sections prepares us to incorporate the checklist in our lives and get the results we have been looking for. This checklist is not a magic wand. That's important for me to state upfront. It's not the holy grail and it does not work if you and I don't work with it. That does not mean that it won't help you get results like those achieved by myself, my father, and the many men and women who have used this exact checklist to drop 20, 30, and even 40 pounds. But, remember, weight loss is not the only goal we have with this checklist. It's about empowering you to both lose weight and keep it off. As I stated earlier in the book, the world does not have a weight loss problem. People lose weight all the time. The issue is weight maintenance. The ability to lose weight and maintain that weight loss is what this checklist will help you with.

As I thought about maintenance, I searched for something that we could all relate to that requires maintenance. What can our bodies be compared to? The idea of a car came to mind. A car has many parts like our bodies do. A car requires maintenance like we do. When you bring your car to the shop, they have a CHECKLIST that they follow regularly to make sure that your car is the best it can possibly be so you're completely safe on the road and can trust the vehicle you're driving. After all, a poorly maintained car puts lives at risk. Our bodies are no different. If we are not able to maintain a healthy weight, we put our lives at risk too. With top car companies producing upwards of 10 million cars a year, you can understand why having a process-oriented approach is so important. The checklist we are about to dive into is that process-oriented approach.

The checklist consists of 8 daily elements that we need to focus on to help us get towards our health and fitness goals and ultimately transform our bodies. Each of the 8 elements are important and you will find as you go through with this that some parts are far more challenging for some people than others. For example, for me, resistance training is not a challenge at all. After all, I have 14 years of experience as a powerlifter, so that is something that is quite familiar to me. The sleeping part, as you will see, was my weakness.

The essential aspect of this checklist is that it's something you can easily tailor for your specific needs. No two people are alike when it comes to their exact lifestyles, but these fundamental elements are at the core of every successful health and fitness transformational program.

The daily 8 in this checklist are:

1. 7.5 hours of sleep
2. Track Your Food
3. 5k Steps
4. See Your Goal
5. Eat More Protein
6. Hydrate
7. Weigh In
8. Assess Your Wins

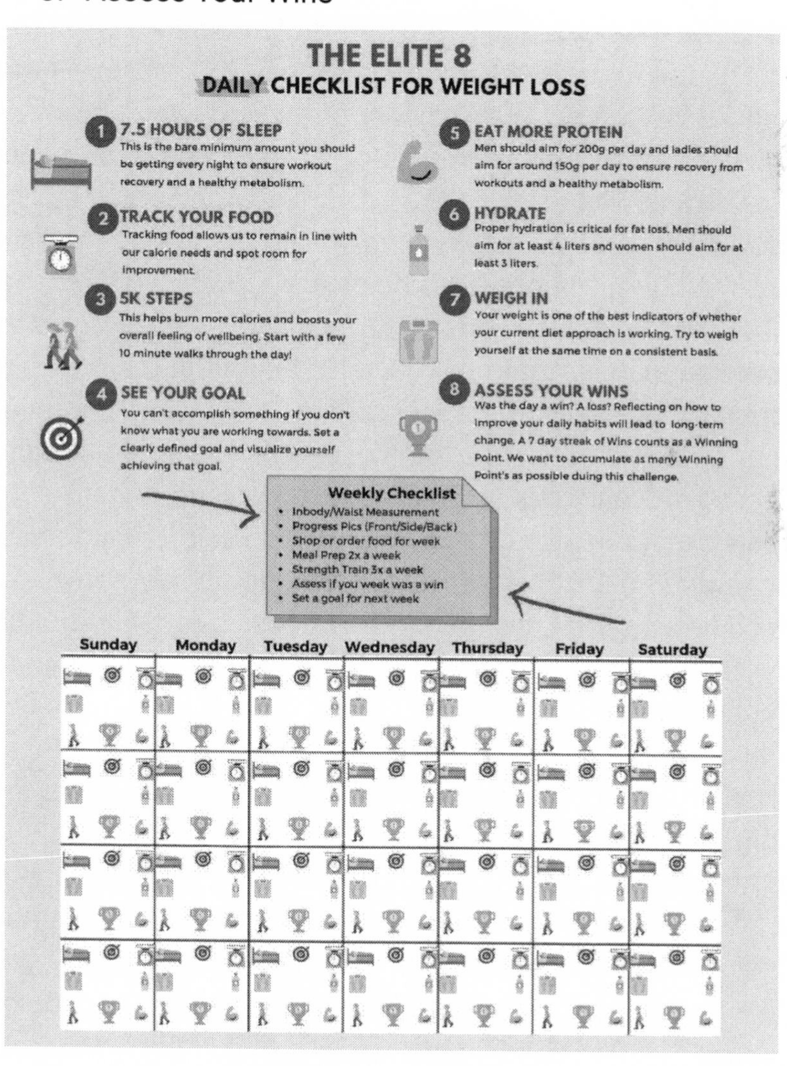

We will dive into each element of the checklist so you fully understand how it is best utilized to meet your goals. For starters, this checklist is daily! There is a weekly checklist you can see in the middle of the image, but we will start with the daily checklist for weight loss. Now, I know for some people the idea of a daily checklist can be overwhelming, especially as you are starting out. The purpose of this checklist is to make sure you know where you are going. We know that life happens and sometimes you might miss a thing or two every now and then. You do not have to beat yourself up when this happens. The best thing you can do is bounce right back. The goal is for us to win more times than we lose. In a 7 day span, if we can see the majority of those days go down as wins, you're well on your way to seeing success with your overall goal. The checklist also doubles as an accountability tool where you can check to make sure you are on the right track. All of this information helps to empower you to know what your next directions need to be so you can arrive at your destination (that goal we talked about in the previous chapter). One quick tip about getting more wins: the more your goal means to you the more likely you will make the necessary sacrifices to meet your goal. Remember how I shared with you in the introduction that I would get bad sleep, wake up in pain, and was not able to do regular activities? In addition to that, my grandfather passing away made me look within to what example I was setting and I resolved to not be someone who simply preaches to others how to live a healthy lifestyle. It was that realization and my desire to share what I have learned with you that drove me to get the daily 8 done on my checklist more times than not. Do you remember your goal? Do you remember why it's important to you? If you don't or forgot it, take a moment, put the book down, and revisit the answer to those questions. Why you do something is just as important as to what you are doing.

Troubleshooting The Checklist

For each step from the daily checklist, write some reflections on your current habits and what you will need to do to improve and check off those items!

For each item answer below: Are you hitting daily minimum? If not, what is one simple thing you can start doing to move yourself towards hitting it. If yes, what is something you can do to enhance or stay consistent with your performance?

- 7.5 Hours of Sleep:

____

____

- Track Your Food:

____

____

- 5k Steps:

____

____

- See Your Goal:

____

____

- Eat More Protein:

___

___

- Hydrate:

___

___

- Weigh-In:

___

___

- Assess Your Wins

___

___

7.5 Hours of Sleep

Let's dive into the first item on the checklist: 7.5 hours of sleep. This ties in with our recovery, something we will be talking about in more detail in the next chapter. For now, though, know that sleep is a key component to everything else we are going to be doing throughout this journey. It is my finding that 7.5 hours of sleep minimum is a good benchmark when it comes to getting the proper rest needed to get the best results with any body transformation program. For more advanced athletes, sometimes upwards of nine hours of sleep is necessary for full recovery. If you are not able to hit 7.5 hours of sleep at minimum, naps might be your best friend. I would suggest against taking them in the middle of the day but a 30, 60, or even 90 minute nap can do wonders for your recovery.

Track Your Food

You've heard the saying that "abs are made in the kitchen" or "you are what you eat"? Well, there is some truth to that. But for the sake of this book, the big thing you need to know about tracking your food is that we cannot manage what we do not measure. It's going to be nearly impossible to make the changes you need to have sustainable weight loss if you are not tracking what you are eating. To track your food, we recommend using the MyFitnessPal app.

5k Steps

Being active is a big part of this process. Remember, when I gained a ton of weight in my journey, it was from the lack of activity. To help with being and staying active, I recommend 5,000 steps daily. The MyFitnessPal app can also calculate your steps and help you keep track. It's important to note that these steps are in addition to your training. When I was active in the past I was lifting, but the 5,000 steps was not part of my routine. Therefore, I was not getting the cardiovascular work that I need to have as part of my regular routine. Your 5,000 steps can come in a variety of ways. You're not limited to just walking. You might want to go on a hike and combine being out in nature as part of getting your 5,000 steps. You can also go on a bike ride. Whatever you do, the goal here is to get in some cardio that amounts to 5,000 steps.

See Your Goal

In the previous chapter, we talked about the value of setting a goal and how it's like entering the destination in a GPS. This is something you want to see every single day. For example, when I had my goal of wanting to weigh under 200 pounds and have 10% body fat by October 3rd, I made sure it was something I saw every single day. Place your goal somewhere you will see it everyday. I placed mine on my fridge. Every time I went to get some water or prepare to eat, I would see my goal right there in front of me. Do the same with your goal.

Eat More Protein

It almost goes without saying how important protein is. Protein is the building block of muscle mass, so you'll want to make sure you eat more of it. Most people do not eat enough protein, so we're going to aim in general to take it up a notch. The amount of protein you'll need to consume will be tied to how much you weigh. We will break that down later on in the book when we address nutrition. For now, note that eating protein is key to maintaining muscle mass and building a healthy metabolism.

Hydrate

In a similar effort to eating protein for an improved metabolism, you are going to want to make sure you are getting enough water. Not only is it important for flushing your body of toxins, but it's also great for keeping those cravings at bay. For most people, thirst is often confused with hunger. While we are feeling hungry, the reality is we may be dehydrated and in need of water. We'll talk more about staying hydrated and outline some tactical approaches we can take to make sure that we give our body the hydration that it needs.

Weigh In

There are many schools of thoughts when it comes to weighing yourself. There is the thought that weighing yourself everyday can be problematic, but there are also great benefits to weighing yourself daily. Many people get flustered with weighing themselves everyday because of daily fluctuations that can leave them feeling defeated with their efforts. Remember, we are weighing ourselves with the sole focus to track overall progress. For the work we are doing in this book, we suggest weighing yourself first thing in the morning after you use the bathroom, but while you are still fasted (before you eat anything). You can also do a weekly average to get a better read on your weight.

Assess Your Wins

Last on the daily checklist is assessing your wins. What was the day? A win? A loss? You want to use this step as a moment of reflection so you can successfully know how your journey is going and be able to make tweaks along the way. If you're able to do every point on the checklist, you get a win. Do it for an entire week and you get a point.

Troubleshooting Daily Habits

- What is your goal and why is it important to you?

____

____

- Which items on the checklist are you currently reflecting on in your life?

___

___

- Rate which habits are hardest, of medium difficulty, or easier for you to maintain overall. You can put them in columns below.
- Hard Medium Easy

___

___

- Focus on the items that you are furthest away from accomplishing first. List them out below. Consider that the thing which you may identify as furthest away may not actually be the most difficult habit for you to maintain. Rather, it is possible that it could be something easier for you to accomplish, but simply neglected from your focus. Think about what needs to move most. In which respect are you furthest from the minimum?

___

___

- In the space below, sketch out a normal daily schedule for you to meet these goals! Write out both a typical work/weekday, off-day/weekend, if necessary. Include everything from when you wake up till when you go to sleep. It does not have to be hard and fast, but you want to envision how and when you will practically accomplish each thing.

____

____

____

____

____

____

____

____

____

____

____

____

For an example to help you out, I have done the same roughly below. Don't just try and copy my schedule, though! It is specialized for my situation and body, as yours should be for you. I have included in parentheses the corresponding checklist items.

6:00 AM: wake up and weigh-in (healthy sleep, weigh-ins)

6:30 AM: Have 1stphorm protein w/ oats, drink 1 liter of water (tracking, protein, hydration)

7:00 AM: 30 mins of steady state cardio (steps)

7:30 AM-8:45 AM: Do resistance training workout, drink 1 liter water throughout (weekly strength training, hydration)

8:45 AM: Have post-workout meal of shrimp and rice

(tracking, protein intake)

9:00 AM: Coaching/Work

10:30-11:00 AM: Finish daily steps (cardio)

11:30-12:00 PM: Have a meal of Piedmontese lean beef, spinach, carrots, white potatoes, drink 1 liter of water. See my goal when I go to the fridge. (tracking, protein, hydration, see your goal)

12:00-3:00 PM: Run errands, complete work, rest, etc.

2:00-3:00 PM: Have meal of salmon, asparagus, drink 1 liter of water (tracking, protein, hydration)

4-8 PM: Coaching/Work

Usually by the afternoon, I am able to assess whether a day is a win or not. Then, I try to make up for what I am missing before bed. I have an alarm at 8:15 PM to remind me to wind down for bed. This allows me to get 7 ½ - 9 hours of sleep a night, depending on whether I am training for a contest or not. With this general schedule, if I am in bed by 9 PM, I could get 9 hours of sleep. Again, your schedule will be very different!

Weekly checklist

Now that we've gotten through the daily checklist, let's dive into the weekly checklist. As we shared earlier, by having this much emphasis on what is happening on this daily, weekly scale, you'll be able to stay on top of things and monitor your progress. This ensures success by allowing us to have a malleable plan. You do not want to unintentionally arrive confused at an undesired destination because you simply followed a static, one-size-fits-all plan and did not make necessary adjustments.

InBody Measurement/Waist Measurement

The Inbody is a machine that measures your body fat. It's an incredible machine that some gyms have. We've used it to get accurate readings for our clients so they are aware of where they are on a week to week basis. Not all gyms have this machine, so, to supplement, you can take weekly waist measurements. Like our daily weigh-ins, the purpose of this is tracking. We want to measure our progress. Sometimes the scale does not tell us all that is happening when it comes to our progress, so this is an additional metric to track our weight loss journey. I've seen many times the scale not move for a few days only to see the waist measurements and/or the body fat measurements tell a different story. This is a way to make sure that we remain encouraged through the journey and have an accurate depiction of how we are doing.

Progress Pictures

Like the Inbody/waist measurements, taking progress pictures allows us to visualize the results over time with our bodies. When taking progress pictures, take a photo of yourself from the front, the side, and the back. We want to do this on a weekly basis to consistently track our progress. A pro-tip is to use the same lighting, same amount of clothes, and the same type of clothes. You want it to look as similar to the previous photo as possible. The only thing that should change is our bodies themselves. Sometimes putting on different clothes will make it hard to see the progress that was made, so we want to keep everything about the process as consistent as possible without having any other factors impact our tracking.

Shop/Order Food

Am I the only one that struggles to eat right? Have you realized how much easier it is to eat the wrong foods when you don't have the right foods around? This is why this action item makes the list. To ensure that you are eating the right foods, you need to have the right foods around. This can be accomplished either by going out and shopping for the food or ordering the food. Either way, being intentional about this process will make it a lot easier to do meal prep. We'll talk more about meal prep later in the book, but my recommendation for meal prep is doing it twice a week. I personally like doing it on Sundays and Wednesdays.

Strength Training 3x/week

In the daily checklist we talked about eating more protein so that we can have the building blocks for building and maintaining muscle mass. Now comes the part that helps us build those muscles up. You're going to strength train three times a week. It can be any combination of days, but they should be every other day, if at all possible. It could be Monday, Wednesday, Friday or it could be Tuesday, Thursday, and Saturday. Whatever combination you use, just know we need resistance training in our journey.

Assess If The Week Was A Win

Like the daily checklist, we want to identify if we earned a win for the week. Measuring whether the week was a win or a loss helps us with the next step on this list which is setting a goal for the next week. The goal is to develop a rhythm and make daily actions on the checklist into our new habits. This will allow you to have some auto-pilot effects when it comes to the things you need to do consistently and repeatedly to get the results you desire.

Set A Goal For Next Week

Once you have done some reflection on how you did daily and weekly with regards to your wins and losses, then you can plan for what the goal is going to be for the next week. We always want to have a destination. A journey without a destination cannot advance. With many other programs, our destination is not clearly set which leads to a setback in our weight loss journey. This is why we shared earlier in the book the value of having short and long term goals and being able to track yourself along the way with these checklist items. It's a lot easier to plan goals when you know what has been working and what has not been working. We cannot do that, however, if we are not keeping track, measuring our progress, and then making the additions or necessary improvements to keep the train on the tracks. Knowing how much you weigh on a daily basis, how many calories you're consuming, how much water you're drinking, and the number of steps you've taken are all data points to help us fuel our weight loss journey.

Troubleshooting Weekly Habits

As we did before with the daily checklist, for each weekly item, write some reflections on your current habits and what you will need to do to improve and check off those points!

- InBody Measurement/Waist Measurement

____

____

- Progress Pictures

____

____

- Shop/Order Food

____

____

- Strength Training 3x/week

____

____

- Assess If The Week Was A Win

____

____

- Set A Goal For Next Week

____

____

Now, once again, sketch out how you would tackle each item over a normal week.

For reference, here is some of what I do:
Strength Training Sessions: Sunday/Monday/

Wednesday/Thursday

Grocery Shopping: Tuesday Mid-day

Meal Prep: Wednesday + Over weekend, if necessary

In-Body or Waist Measurements: Thursday (if you have a treat meal on the weekends, you will be normalized by Thursday)

Progress Pics: Saturday

____

____

____

____

____

____

Checklist Walk Through

Now that you know the elements of both the daily and weekly checklist, I'm going to go through an example of my food intake log, so you can see how to begin incorporating these habits into your life. It's said that we learn better when we are shown things and not just told them, so this is the showing portion of the program :-)

[Coach Gaglione Food Intake From February 2nd, 2020]

EDIT < Sun, Feb 2 >

Calories Remaining

2,640	-	2,664	+	93	=	69
Goal		Food		Exercise		Remaining

Breakfast Carbs 27% · Fat 22% · Protein 50%	2,664
Asparagus Spears Asparagus Spears, 4 container (6 spears ea.)	72
beef 93% lean bjs wholesale, 24 oz 113g	1,020
Cage Free Egg Whites Kirkland Signature, 1 container (460 gs ea.)	250
Casein Protein - Chocolate Peanut Butter Optimum Nutrition, 4 heaping scoop (33g)	480
whole fresh Strawberries Wish Farms, ½ container (16.00 oz)	72
Light String Cheese Frigo Cheeseheads, 3 Piece (24g)	150
Sprouted Brown Sticky Rice Annie Chun's™, 1 Tray (180g)	280
Sticky White Rice Bowl	

Above is an image of some of my food intake from February 2nd, 2020. You can see everything's in here. You will notice that I did not input things meal by meal. This can be different for each person. For some, putting every single meal in there may be a great place to start. In fact, I would suggest starting there and then over time you will develop a habit where it becomes automatic and you may not have to jot down every single meal. This, again, is not about perfection but about sustainable progression towards our goals. On this occasion, I forgot to input my meals ahead of time, which is why it is not a complete record. If you fail to plan, you plan to fail. If you can input this ahead of time before you are eating, it's easier to follow along versus having to improvise when you're hungry.

Let us jump back to what we see in the image above. It says I had 24 ounces of beef that day. Before you judge me and assume I live like a viking from premodern times, I did not eat that all at once. I spread the ounces throughout the day. Sometimes I'll have two 12 ounce portions and other times I'll have six ounces pre-workout, another six ounces post-workout, and then a separate meal with 12 ounces. For those who think this is a lot of beef, it's important to remember that we need to eat more protein and also this is tied to how much you weigh.

For breakfast, I would eat my string cheese with my egg whites for flavor. I would then have berries by themselves around my workout time. Then, I would have asparagus later in the day with some lean protein. Here it says 93% lean. At the time of writing this book I'm using 96%. It was a progression as my goals began to change. I started off at 90% before getting to the 96%. As I shared with you earlier, as your goals change so must your approach to getting there. What got you to where you were won't get you to where you want to go, but, with the checklist and the tracking, I'm able to make those changes as needed because I understand the fundamentals. To round out my protein, you can see I had eggs (normally I have whole eggs, just didn't on this particular day) and then made some casein pudding to complete my protein intake. Now, if you look at the image below which displays my daily macronutrients, you can see that I had over 300 grams of protein per day, my fats are under 80 grams, and my carbs are under 200 while my calories are under 3000 on this particular day. My protein represented 50% of my diet. Now, you're not going to start there, but I just want to show an example of the "eat more protein" part from the checklist.

[Coach Gaglione Macronutrients from Feb 2nd, 2020]

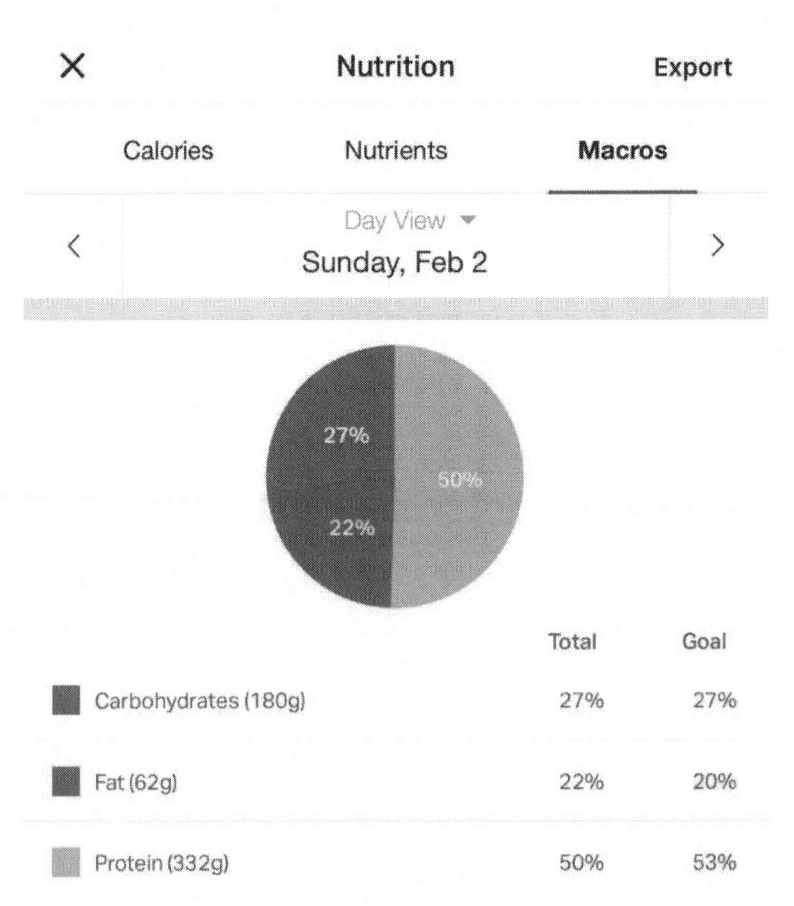

It's a lot easier to make this automatic when you are able to keep the food as similar as possible on a day to day basis. There are ways to tweak the eating for variety like adding different sources and diversifying how you're consuming your greens, your protein, and so on. I will share more on this with you, but remember that you will stay on track longer by maintaining consistency and making the process as convenient as possible in order to minimize stress and error.

If we went through a longer section of my log, you could see that I started to drop my caloric intake a bit as I was looking to drop some weight. You'd also see that I am not perfect. I missed tracking a day that week, even. That would mean a loss when assessing if I earned a win that week. This does not mean it's the end of the world. Simply make the adjustment when setting your goal for the next week. Because we are going to be logging a lot of entries, it happens, but we want to minimize those occurrences as much as possible.

In addition to tracking our food, we also have our weigh-ins as well our steps. When using MyFitnessPal, you can see this information better on your phone than on the computer version.

During the time of the images shown, I weighed about 220 pounds. Then it was holiday time. I purposely bulked up so I could compete in the 242 class. My weight got as heavy as 248. I probably didn't actually track 248 because I was too embarrassed (guilty). I started at about 246. Through my bulking, I experienced a lot of fluctuation. As I got closer and closer to my meets, my weight began to drop. I like to stay about 5-15 pounds away from the weight

I need to be for a meet and then really ramp things up to hit where I need to be.

As you can see, this entire process is not black and white. There is a lot of gray and the actions I take are dependent on what my goals require. The coolest thing about this approach is that I'm the one driving the car towards the destination the whole way through. Since I am tracking all of my habits and my progress, I can make adjustments as necessary. If I notice some traffic on the road, I can pull over, evaluate what is happening, and then get a new set of directions to make sure I am still able to arrive at my destination. The checklist is the key to making sure that I have that power. You now have it too. You can refer to the image and also go to the resources section to contact us for a digital copy. Later in the book, we will go even deeper with each element of the checklist so that you have more specific direction on how to maximize your efforts to complete the 8 daily elements in the context of the weekly approach. We'll be talking about different ways to get your cardio training in, what strength training can look like for you even if you aren't a powerlifter, how to get your protein up, how to prep your meals, and I will offer some practical advice on how to improve your eating habits. Next up, however, is the number one thing that is often overlooked. I overlooked it big time and when I finally got a handle on it, all the dominoes began to fall.

Troubleshooting Daily Nutrition

- What does your daily nutrition look like now? Sketch out, to the best of your memory, what you ate on a recent day. If you're new to tracking, a really good technique is just to take photos of everything you eat and reference later to monitor your habits.

____

____

- Write down your 3 favorite sources of carbs, sources of protein, vegetables, and fruits. For example, my favorites are:
  Carbs: white potatoes, sweet potato, oats
  Protein: lean beef/steak (piedmontese), shrimp, salmon
  Vegetables: spinach, carrots, mushrooms
  Fruits: berries (raspberries, blueberries, strawberries, cranberries), kiwi, oranges

____

____

- Out of these favorite foods, what healthy options can you add to your plan?

____

____

- Reflect on your regular diet, do any foods lead you to overeat, cause digestive stress, or make you feel guilty? Consider limiting your intake of these foods or eliminating them from your diet entirely. For me, bagels fit the bill for all of these things. I'm not going to have just one. I'm going to have five-- and my stomach will be upset after. What food does that to you?

____

____

- How will your specific goals affect your ideal nutrition habits?

____

____

- What is one simple change you can make to improve your nutrition today?

____

____

CHAPTER 4

SLEEP

When it comes to losing weight there are typical things that we normally hear as far as advice goes. We hear statements like:

- You are what you eat
- You cannot out-train a bad diet
- An apple a day keeps the doctor away
- Make sure you eat your greens
- Be active

These are good statements and they are so often repeated because they honestly are solid pieces of advice. The funny thing about cliches is that there is, in fact, a lot of truth to them. Sleep, however, isn't typically the focus of common weight-loss advice. There is no cute saying that has been cycled around time and time again. Perhaps this is why I easily overlooked the impact that sleep could have on my progress in my weight-loss journey.

It's not until more recently that the idea of recovery became as popular as it is today. Many ideas of peak performance started off with an emphasis on just training. It would later evolve to making sure you have your nutrition dialed in to take advantage of the work you were putting in the gym. Now, we often hear that if your recovery is not right, you won't be able to get the most out of the efforts you've put in at the gym.

If the end results of our weight loss journey are going to be good, one thing that can help is having a good start. The start does not begin when you walk into the gym or even when you wake up. The start begins the night before. This is something I wish someone would have told me years ago. Do you know how much agony and frustration I could have avoided with this information? How many easy going mornings I missed out on because I did not know the connection between how my day ended and how my day began? This is why we place sleep first in the daily checklist.

The first step, where it all begins, is by getting our 7.5 hours of sleep. Are you wondering why not just an even 8 hours? Well, it's because our sleep cycles are typically 90 minutes long, not 60 minutes long. Like everything, ideal amounts of sleep can vary. Some people need up to 10 hours of sleep to help with their recovery. This is typically for those who are in a competition phase or if you're looking to get really lean like I did when I was preparing for my bodybuilding show. It's not easy to do, especially being a full-time coach, entrepreneur, and having healthy relationships with family and friends, but it's key. Remembering how your day ends plays an integral role in how your next day begins.

As I was going for my 900 pound squat back in the day, or even doing my 800 pounds squat for different weight classes, I noticed how much adding a 20, 30, or even 90-minute nap helped to accelerate my recovery and allow me to train harder. When I did not have those naps, my energy levels were poor, my productivity was poor, and I was a pest to be around.

So, a basic benchmark for sleep is to get your 7.5 hours. Now, before you tell me about your friend who is great with just 5 hours, note that this is just a generalization that works for most. No one person is all alike. There will be outliers who are able to make 3-5 hours work, but this is not typical. Don't assume that just because you can function at 5 hours of sleep, you should. I've found 7.5 hours to be a good consensus for the majority to test and then adjust as you track the impact it has on your recovery and overall health.

Sleep Study

As I began my journey towards troubleshooting areas that were holding back my weight loss efforts, I reached out to IFBB Bodybuilding and World Record Powerlifter Stan Efferding, along with other colleagues. It was on their recommendation that I got a sleep study done. The people who conducted my sleep study were alarmed at the results. It's never a great sign when those who are administering an exam or study are alarmed. It means that something is off or unusual. The sleep study revealed that my sleep apnea was very bad. When I went to sleep, I was essentially choking on myself. Think about repeatedly choking while you are sleeping. Now, you can imagine why I had a hard time getting quality sleep. Being a weightlifter and having a thick neck did not help my cause either. This meant that my airway was a lot smaller, making it harder to get oxygen. If you have a thick neck, are powerlifter/weightlifter, or if you are just someone who has a hard time feeling rested, even if you do get the "hours of sleep" regularly, a sleep study is definitely worth looking into.

Another suggestion that Stan Efferding brought to my attention was a dream station machine. A dream station machine is a C-PAP machine that can help anyone who has sleep apnea. It's helped me tremendously to get better quality sleep. I believe you can get them at major pharmacies now without needing a prescription. Without getting too technical here or passing myself off as a sleep expert (which I am not), the machine works by applying various amounts of pressure. As I lost the weight, I noticed that I needed less and less pressure than before. I continued to use it every single night and, when we had a loss of power in my area one night, I noticed the difference when I did not use it. My sleep was horrible!

Some other specific things I've done also to help with my sleep quality are using blue light glasses a few hours before bed, performing breathing exercises, and taking cold showers, just to name a few. You'll learn more about the different strategies you can use to improve your sleep quality when we break down the 3 Ts to improving your quality of sleep.

How to improve sleep quality for performance

In order for us to improve our sleep quality, it's important for us to understand the basics of sleep and how our daily lives may inhibit healthy sleeping. It's only by understanding this that we can counterbalance the damage that our current habits have produced which may stop us from getting the best sleep quality we can possibly get.

Long before the invention of electricity, giving us our electric lights, alarm clocks, and now the smartphones that we use for our alarm clocks, our bodies would regulate sleep according to natural light sources and temperature.

Let's look at an example of what sleep was like back then. Before electricity and smartphones came into play, one would see their sleep managed by what time of the day it was. Towards the middle of the day, when the sun is at the highest in the sky, people would tend to be the most alert. This would be around 11:00 AM to Noon, typically. As we made our way to the end of the day, the temperature would begin to drop as the light started to recede. That is when people would start to wind down. When it became completely dark, people would just go to sleep. This is what it was like when there was no electricity or phones. The body has a natural way of figuring stuff out, a natural bio-rhythm, if you will, but modern society ruined all of that for us.

So, you may be wondering, what do we do about it? Well, that is where I'd like to introduce you to the 3 Ts to improving your quality of sleep. Before jumping into each of the three parts, however, it's important that we realize that, like everything written in this book, it's not an overnight process. Everything we are doing in this book is gradual because it allows us to be present to the changes and be able to make tweaks along the way.

I mention this because the same way Rome was not built in a day, neither will revamping our sleep quality be accomplished in a single night. Did you know that a third of your life is spent sleeping? That means if you live to be 100 years old, you will be asleep for the equivalent of 33.33 years. It's not going to be instantaneous to change a third of your life, but with a process and a specific strategy in place, it is very doable to see improvements with your sleep quality which will positively impact other areas of your life like exercising, nutrition, mood, and overall health.

As you can see in the image of the chart below, there are 3 specific components we are going to focus on to improve our quality of sleep.

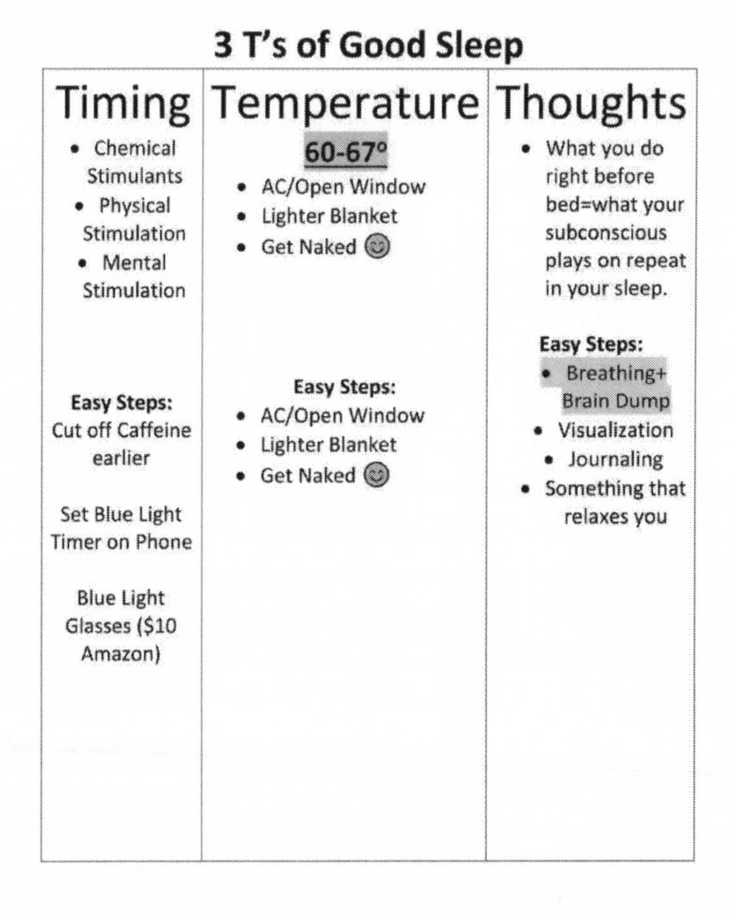

3 T's of Good Sleep

Timing	Temperature	Thoughts
• Chemical Stimulants • Physical Stimulation • Mental Stimulation	60-67° • AC/Open Window • Lighter Blanket • Get Naked 😊	• What you do right before bed=what your subconscious plays on repeat in your sleep.
Easy Steps: Cut off Caffeine earlier Set Blue Light Timer on Phone Blue Light Glasses ($10 Amazon)	**Easy Steps:** • AC/Open Window • Lighter Blanket • Get Naked 😊	**Easy Steps:** • Breathing+ Brain Dump • Visualization • Journaling • Something that relaxes you

Timing

The first T we will discuss is timing. When working on the different Ts, I suggest that you focus on one for some amount of time, say, a month, and then, once you have a good grasp on it, move onto the next. And just so you do not feel overwhelmed, you do not have to tackle the entire column in the chart at once. You can do one bullet point at a time.

For the purpose of this section, when we talk about timing we are referring to the timing of the things that you're doing and the stimulation that you're putting into your body. One example of something you could be putting to your body is caffeine. I'm a caffeine junkie. How about you? Are you a frequent caffeine user? Caffeine can come in many different forms: coffee, energy drinks, and even teas contain caffeine. All of these introduce a chemical stimulant into our bodies.

Physical activity is another form of stimulation. If you're someone that likes to work out later in the evening, maybe after work, that is something that should be considered part of the conversation when we are talking about timing. For some people, working out later in the day knocks them right out to sleep, while for others it serves almost like a chemical stimulant like coffee, preventing them from getting to sleep right away.

Then we have mental stimulation. What does that look like? Imagine someone who decides their bedtime is 10:00 PM, yet right before at 9:59 PM they go to bed answering stressful emails. Many might think the minute you stop doing the activity that your body is at rest, but that is not the case. It's not like an on/off switch. Think about it like the pre-modern times where light is receding through the day gradually and the temperature, likewise, is slowly changing throughout the day. It's not instant. Rather than an on/off switch, the better comparison is to those light dimmers that you might have in a living room or dining room. Your mind and body are more so a dial than an on/off switch.

Because these stimulating effects are not instantaneous, your health and understanding of your body will benefit from taking a tapering approach to them accordingly. Take, for example, caffeine. Did you know that caffeine has a half life of about 6 hours? This means that if you had 200 mg of caffeine in one of your beverages, you will still have 100 mg of caffeine in your system 6 hours later! That's insane, isn't it? We're over here wondering, "if I had coffee back at 2 PM, how come I'm still feeling like I have some caffeine still in my body at 8 PM?" Well, now you know why. It is due to the half life of caffeine. This is why I have a cut-off point after which I do not consume caffeine at all. If I am trying to be asleep by 9 or 10 PM, I know that I need to have my last drink containing caffeine at around 12 or 1 PM to make sure it's almost all out of my body by the time I am looking to get to bed. Now, every day isn't the same, so I might need it a little bit later in the day due to meetings or other circumstances, but on average I try not to go past 1 PM. As such, I am able to make sure my sleep is not compromised, which is especially important because I understand how poor sleep can hinder my recovery and my energy levels the next day.

What is your cut-off point going to be? Start with your time of sleep (goal) and work backwards. Remember, you need a minimum of 7.5 hours, so start there and work backwards so you can know when best to cut off your caffeine.

Our quality of sleep can also be improved by applying this tapering approach to our exposure to light. Remember that light communicates to our bodies that it is still day time. This can make it harder to fall asleep or get good quality sleep. When it comes to your bedroom, you'll often hear that you want to have blinds that can block out any light from the window and to make sure your room is dark so that it is easier to sleep. I personally use eye masks in addition to those suggestions to try to keep the room as dark as possible.

We also get light from our televisions, cell phones, and tablets. This light is not best for our eyes when we are looking to go to sleep. This is why you hear a lot of people say that you should stop using your devices by a certain time if you want to get good quality sleep. There are certain things that have worked for me when it comes to limiting my brain's exposure to light. Setting a blue-light timer on my phone is one of them. Blue light basically tells our bodies that it's not time to go to sleep yet, therefore we stay awake following exposure to it. I set my blue-light time to 6:00 PM. This makes my phone look a little more yellow. It does not ruin the quality of the image but it does help me to ensure that my mind is not stimulated such that I won't be able to shut my body down. I also have this feature installed on my laptop using a blue light app. Sometimes we bring work home or have to put in a few extra hours on the computer, so having an app like this allows me to be able to make the transition from work to sleep more smoothly. If you are not able to get any of these apps, there are blue light filters you can find online that can help minimize the mental stimulation.

One more tool that I want to share with you are plastic blue light glasses for when you are watching television. They are super affordable at $10 on Amazon and help again to minimize the mental stimulation of blue light. I know it's a lot harder to kick the Netflix and chill habit than it is to just throw on some blue light glasses, so this is a good option to make it a little bit easier on your body.

I started with this T because it's usually the hardest one to change. I believe this has a lot to do with social norms. You open up your Instagram and you see, for example, everything is about coffee this, cold brew that, nitro this, and so that automatic, subconscious suggestion makes you think that you need to have that too. Also, with our grind culture where we praise constant productivity, the idea of relaxation and rest is often minimized or even demonized. That's not even to mention the ubiquity of screens!

Before even making any changes to your sleep timing, a good place to start is by just becoming aware of what your mental, physical, and chemical stimulation is like. Then, you can make tweaks to one habit, see how that goes, and then add on as you see fit. Again, everything is about progression, having full control, and driving the car to your destination. You're the driver.

Temperature

The next T is temperature. Everyone has their preferences when it comes to temperature and there have been a ton of studies that suggest what is best. Personally, I'm a fan of sleeping in an icebox. I'll often sleep with the air conditioning on or, at the very least, have a fan on to make sure that the room is cool. According to research, the ideal temperature for sleeping is 60 to 67 degrees Fahrenheit. Compare this to our normal body temperature which is 98.7 degrees Fahrenheit. This reflects conditions in premodern times where, as the sunlight would fade and the night would come, temperatures would cool and indicate to the body that it's coming close to nighttime and we should lower the plane, metaphorically speaking, to land and come to a complete rest.

Out of all three of the Ts, I find this one to be a far easier adjustment. We can easily make a room cooler by opening a window, turning on the AC, or having a fan circulating. Some people keep cool by using only a light blanket and going to sleep with no clothes at all. Interestingly, a lot of studies have shown that not changing anything except for sleeping without clothes allows your body to regulate its temperature a lot more easily. So, even if you didn't change the temperature of your room, just not wearing clothing has its benefits. Just leave those cool pajamas off to the side. Of course, if it's an icebox one night, by all means throw some clothes on or throw a blanket over yourself. Other easy adjustments I like to make include not wearing socks, replacing a shirt with a tank, or trading pants for shorts. All of these suggestions help your body regulate the temperature better, so you can get the quality of sleep you need.

Thoughts

The last T stands for our thought processes. I usually like to leave this one for last because the thought process conversation is the one that typically is met with the most resistance. "Your brain is sabotaging your sleep" is something that most people do not want to hear. No one wants to be told they are thinking potentially unhealthy thoughts and that this is why their sleep sucks and they aren't able to find success with their weight loss/body transformation journey. It's received as a personal attack versus the more physical adjustments in temperature or timing.

Evaluating your thought process requires a lot more introspection, which means a little bit more work than is involved with the previous two Ts. If you have not done the first two Ts, I would suggest doing those first before diving into this one, unless you just enjoy taking challenging things head on. Knocking those two Ts first might give you the momentum you need to be able to handle this T.

This T is more suited for those who have found their sleep is destroyed by stress, especially emotional stress. That is where the issue of our thought processes shows up the most. When we go to bed with troubling thoughts, we are programming our subconscious minds to broadcast them on repeat throughout the night. Have you ever watched a movie and then had a bizarre dream with bits and pieces of that movie? Perhaps you watched a horror movie and then you had a dream where you're being chased by bigfoot or something? Whatever you expose your brain to before going to sleep has a greater likelihood of participating in your sleep.

A strategy you can use to help with this is replacing the activities you do before going to bed. One of the activities I do in particular are breathing exercises. Breathing exercises allow my body to calm down. It's like lowering the flame under some food while cooking or dimming that light like we talked about before. Another thing you can do is journaling or using some visualization exercises before going to bed. Now, I know this might seem like some new-age stuff and I'm not necessarily pushing that agenda, but visualization and journaling have been recommended by so many people for a reason. They work!

When I mention journaling, it does not necessarily mean that you give your diary a name, write "today was hard", and that's it. There is a thought leader named Craig Ballantyne who had a great suggestion on what to do in your journal that I really liked. He called it "brain dumping". It's an opportunity for you to just jot down everything that is on your mind: the good, the bad, the stuff you have to do tomorrow, what happened to you that day, what you cannot seem to stop thinking about. Put it all down. I recommend doing this on paper and not typing on a device. Remember, if we are able to minimize our exposure to blue light while doing these activities, it's only going to help us regulate more effectively and help us get better quality sleep. I like brain dumping in particular because it allows me a place to log my thoughts and not have them take up space in my mind. It also helps if I ever have to go back to see how or what I was thinking last week or two months ago. If I was in a great mood two weeks ago, I can see what my thoughts were like before going to bed at the time and strive to repeat whatever I did that particular day. Combining that with MyFitnessPal can give me so much data and information to help me continue to make big progress on my journey.

What if you're not the journaling type? Simply choose an activity that calms you. For some of you, that might be knitting. If knitting calms you, do that. It does not require anything that would give you blue light and you can easily do it in the room you sleep in, if you want to. Maybe you want to read an entertaining fiction book instead of watching television, so that you can get your Netflix-type entertainment without exposing yourself to blue light. Whatever the activity might be, when it comes to minimizing your mental stimulation, anything that can calm and relax you would be a great thing to add to your sleeping repertoire.

To conclude this chapter, I want to recap that no one's sleep is ever going to be perfect, but if we can mitigate the damage of modern life, you're going to see a massive improvement. Remember that you might not need every single technique presented here. For me, my room is always an icebox, so that covers the temperature. Personally, I need to work on the thought process column. For you, it might be the timing. It might be all three, but I don't want you to look at the chart and think, "Wow, I need to fix 27 things because I'm really broken."

It might just be one or two things that you really need to dial in. Now, you might be wondering about supplements. Are there any we can take to help with our sleep? I purposely left that out in this section because most of us are able to regulate our bodies without needing to use external stimulants to do so. I'd rather you be empowered to work from within and be able to control your body yourself than become reliant on supplementation.

So, there you have it. We talked about getting your 7.5 hours minimum, why it's important, and outlined the practical strategies that can help make sure you get the best quality of sleep you can. This will position us to be able to focus on the last two sections which every program discusses, exercise and nutrition.

Troubleshooting Sleep

- How much sleep did you get last night? Was your sleep interrupted? Was it restful? How did you feel when you woke up?

____

____

____

____

- Write, on average, when you go to sleep and when you wake up? How consistent are you with these times? If not consistent, what is one simple change you can make to improve the consistency of your sleep schedule?
- Which "T" of healthy sleep is most difficult for you? Which are you doing on a regular basis already? Which would be easy to improve?

____

____

____

____

- Write 3 steps you will take to improve your sleep. For example, if you're a caffeine drinker, what will your cut-off point be?

To give an example from my life, I have an alarm at 8:15 PM to remind me to start getting to bed. I use blue light glasses, make sure my room is dark and cool, and I get away from electronics. Then, I use my CPAP machine and an eye mask to help improve my sleep quality. If I am having trouble sleeping, I often take a hot or cold shower. Either can be relaxing and bring your body temperature down. If you are constantly waking or snoring, you may consider conducting a sleep study. These tips would not be able to fully correct that type of difficulty, but it could be a real lynchpin in your progress to treat it.

____

____

____

____

CHAPTER 5

5K STEPS

"A body in motion stays in motion".

Have you ever heard this quote before?

This quote is one that I can resonate with. Typically, those who have health issues are those who live a sedentary lifestyle, one where they are not moving at all. Our bodies were made to move. The question becomes, what movements should we be doing? At what intensity should we be performing these movements?

In this chapter, we are going to talk about the various activities we can do to remain active and allow us to check that activity level box on our daily checklist. As it states on the checklist, we want to get 5,000 steps daily. Now, for some that might sound like a lot, for some it might sound like too little, and others will need to learn how to even track that stuff and make it part of their current lifestyle. We'll address all of this and then some in this chapter. By the end of this chapter, you will know what your exercising should look like in order for you to have sustainable success in reaching the health and fitness goals that you mapped out earlier in the goal setting section of the book.

For starters, why 5k in steps? I'll be honest that, at first, the thought of 5k in steps did not make sense to me. Coming from a powerlifting background and being a high school wrestler, the idea of taking steps did not sound intense enough to me. I was looking at stuff like pulling a pick-up truck or pushing a sled that weighs a ton as good activity. As I evaluated the habits of people who were able to not only lose weight but keep it off for a long period of time, I realized there was a key component about activity levels. That key component was STAYING ACTIVE in a consistent manner. Have you seen athletes who performed at a very high level and then, once they stopped competing, they were not able to maintain that level of fitness? I was guilty of this when I was in high school before transitioning into powerlifting. My activity level while wrestling allowed me to be a part of the 198 weight class. Once I no longer was in wrestling, however, my activity level began to shift. I was active less and less and, well, you know how the story goes. I became 340+ pounds.

The most important elements for us when it comes to activity levels are consistency and sustainability. That is where the habit of 5k steps comes in. I cannot tell you how many times I've read in magazines or heard stories about people who were able to drop weight and keep it off by performing some activity that on the surface might not seem like the most intense thing. Their secret sauce was they did it consistently and were able to sustain that level of activity. This is why the 5k in steps makes our daily checklist. It creates the foundation to be able to not only be active, but stay active.

IFBB bodybuilding pro Stan Efferding, who I mentioned earlier, recommends three 10 minute walks a day. Does that sound doable? Pretty manageable, right? Do 10 minutes here, 10 minutes there, and then wrap up the day with 10 minutes. For my part, I recommend 5,000 steps because sometimes it's not so easy to have 3 appointments on your schedule scattered like that for 10 minute walks. The concept is the same though. Get your butt moving and make it something that is not intense.

Since walking 5,000 steps is not so intense, we can do it every single day. That INCLUDES rest days. So, even on your "day off", you are still walking those 5,000 steps. Remember the opening quote, "a body in motion stays in motion". Let's keep those results moving and not let them go stale by continuing to stay active.

When I was getting ready to compete in my bodybuilding show, cardio was big for me. So much so that I was doing it seven days a week. For the sake of variety, my steps did not just come in the form of walking though. If you're someone who likes variety in your routine, note you can get your steps in many different ways. I would get a lot of my steps on the Stair Master. The important part of the cardio we are doing throughout this program is that you can sustain your efforts and be consistent with it. For many, the Stair Master is very intense, but there are ways to minimize the intensity. When I was doing the Stair Master, I kept the speed that I was doing it very similar to the speed I would walk. I did not have to walk faster. The intensity adjustment to make it a little more challenging was already embedded into the machine, as it was like I was walking up a hill. You can also do this by walking on an incline on the treadmill, if you want to push yourself a little bit but still monitor your intensity. This isn't a beat your body up session, especially since we have to do it everyday. The aim is to accomplish the minimum that you can do while still giving your body what it needs.

Other Ways To Get Your 5,000 Steps

If you're like me, you still want to feel like that CrossFit top notch athlete, so maybe you want to put a little flavor into logging your 5,000 steps. Here are some things you can do to tickle your fancy in that regard.

First, you can use a weight vest when you are walking. A weight vest will make it a little more challenging, but not so much that you feel like you will need extra time to recover and not be able to do it every day. Some people like to use a backpack with weight in it. That is an option too if you do not have a weight vest, but be mindful that because the weight is on your back it could cause some back issues for those who already have issues with their backs.

Another tool you can use to get your 5,000 steps is pushing or dragging a sled. Again, it's a little bit more challenging, but it gives you something to work towards. You can start off walking with zero strength and work your way to adding some light strength to make it different and challenging. A prowler is also an option, if your training facility has access to one or if you already have it at your disposal.

The last two tools I enjoy using to get low intensity cardio are rowers and assault bikes. These two tools allow me to involve my entire body and I can easily do them without concern for injury. They also stimulate the athlete in me who wants to do something that is still technical in nature but without having to become a master at it.

What about Jogging to get to 5k In Steps?

When it comes to jogging, especially for those who are starting out with a little more weight, I subscribe to what Will Farrell says in the movie Anchorman: "jogging is kind of like speed limping". LOL. The challenge with jogging for many is maintaining good mechanics. I've found a lot of jogging can beat up your body and can be muscle wasting.

Now, there's certainly a good way to do it. For example, if you are a former track athlete and you want to incorporate some tempo runs and some sprinting at moderate intensities, I think that can certainly be an option. But for the average person, I think just walking is the way to go.

Overall, the goal is to make sure that we are able to get 20-30 minutes per day of work that is low intensity in nature. A good way to gauge if the work is low intensity is if you can do nasal breathing only. If you are able to do your work without having to breathe through your mouth, that will let you know that you are not doing something that is too intense. This ensures that you have the energy you need for the work later on in this chapter, strength training, which we will be doing three times per week as laid out in our weekly checklist.

The Other Type of Cardio

We've talked a lot about low intensity cardio and the significance it has towards us being able to have consistency and sustainability with our activity levels. There is another type of cardio that I'd like to address here and that is high intensity cardio and the difference between low intensity and high intensity cardio. I believe what's often missing when it comes to cardio and seeing stagnation in our training efforts is a lack of awareness concerning the different types of training we can do, the pros and cons of those techniques, and how best to implement them into our current lifestyles while adjusting them to meet our specific goals. Armed with this information, we will be able to make better decisions on how to keep moving forward with our training.

The first thing worth mentioning is that not all cardio is created equally. If it all were the same, there would be no need for the distinction between low and high intensity. We talked earlier about the benefits of low intensity cardio. Since we are able to do it everyday, it's easier to be consistent with it and it's something we can be sustainable at doing because it requires less recovery time. There are, however, drawbacks to low intensity cardio that are worth mentioning.

Low intensity cardio workouts typically are on the longer side of duration time compared to high intensity cardio. For example, we talked earlier about having to do 20-30 minutes of low intensity cardio like 5,000 steps, or 10 minute walks three times a day. For those who might be pressed for time, maybe you don't have 30 minutes or maybe because the activity becomes so easy, you might have to go to 60 minutes and that might not be feasible for your schedule.

High intensity cardio sessions, however, can be shorter workouts and are more interval based by nature. High intensity cardio, if we were to measure it by our heart rate, is more taxing to our bodies. For those who use heart rate monitors, which I typically do to track my intensity levels when training, high intensity is when you are at greater than 80% of your maximum heart rate. Low intensity is when you are at less than 80% of your maximum heart rate. Being able to maintain greater than 80% of your maximum rate is not something you can sustain for a long time, which is why they are more interval based exercise, meaning that you perform a high effort activity, rest, and then return to the high effort activity. Low intensity is more of a slow and steady approach, which is why you may have heard it referred to as "steady state" cardio.

A good way to think of the difference between the two would be to imagine doing a 100 meter sprint versus running a marathon. A marathon is clearly an activity which takes a longer period of time compared to a 100 meter sprint. A marathon can be 4-5 hours for some, while a 100 meter sprint can be 10-20 seconds.

Tabatas - Interval Training

When speaking of interval training for high intensity cardio, one of my absolute favorite techniques are tabatas. You may have heard of these before. Typically, people use them as a format for some type of circuit training. You may see stuff like Tabata burpees, Tabata kettlebell swings, or Tabata air squats. People have used them in many ways over time and, through various interpretations, have deviated from the original intent of Tabatas. So, I'm going to share with you their original intent so that you can know how best to incorporate them into your workouts to get great benefits.

Tabatas originally were designed to be eight rounds of 20 seconds of work followed by 10 seconds of rest. While performing the eight rounds, if, for example, you got to the seventh round and found your level of performance drop, you would stop the workout altogether and not finish that eighth round. Now, you might be wondering why you would do that. The reason is that the exercise was specifically designed to be done at a specific intensity and, once that goes out the window, it essentially becomes empty work at that point.

The role of performing Tabata is to push yourself to nearly 100%. The reason I specifically share this clarification with you is so you are not left with the perception that you are getting benefits from doing Tabata crunches, for example. Tabatas are designed specifically to be challenging and often involve multiple muscle groups. So, I better not see Tabata Bicep Curls on my social media timeline because I'll be coming for you with the "C'mon" or the "Really" face in the comments section.

Ways to Incorporate Tabatas In Your Training

With Tabatas being essentially 4 minutes in total, there are some really good ways to incorporate them to get a challenging workout. One of my favorite ways is to use the assault bike. The assault bike is great because you are using both your arms and legs and you are really able to tax your body in a way that you cannot use other exercises.

Another goodie is using a rowing machine or a skier machine. Both are total body movements that you can use to go hard and maintain the original intent of performing a Tabata workout.

These are all machines that you can go hard with and have minimal risk to your body.

Warning: If you're someone who is not used to doing cardio, whether you haven't ever done it or you're out of the habit, low intensity, steady state stuff is going to be way safer for beginners.

Remember how I talked about the sprints earlier and how they are more high intensity? There was someone I knew who was a trainer and he was in great shape. One day, he took one of his clients to the track to do sprints and decided to join the person who happened to be in varsity track as a junior in their last sprint for the day. I received a text from him telling me, "I just tore my hamstring". I immediately responded, "how did you do that?" That's when he shared with me that he joined one of his clients on their last sprint. I share this with you because I want you to be aware at all times about weighing the risk versus the reward. Sprinting was not something that he did nor was it something he worked himself into. When you think about your training and going from low intensity to high intensity, I want you to remember the reward, your goal, and ensure that you gradually work yourself into these things versus just throwing yourself in and risking injury.

That being said, I do not want you to fear performing high intensity cardio. There are clearly benefits to incorporating these techniques, but it's important to be mindful of how they are used. A tool is only as effective as how it's utilized. A hammer is great to hit a nail, but if you are using it to cut a piece of paper, it's not going to get the job done.

Before we get off the high intensity train, I want to share with you an additional benefit you get besides shorter workouts. There is this thing called EPOC (excess post oxygen consumption) that happens when you perform high intensity training. Another way the industry refers to EPOC is the "afterburn effect'. This "afterburn effect" basically means that you benefit by having an elevated metabolism for 24-72 hours when you perform a high intensity workout. This is something you do not get with low intensity cardio. This does not mean you should skip low intensity cardio at all. This is just an additional tool I want you to be mindful of so that, when you want to tweak things with your training or make new goals, you are aware of a technique you can use to increase your efforts and get more bang for your buck.

So, we've talked about getting your 5,000 steps, we talked about low intensity versus high intensity cardio, went down Tabata lane, and discussed how to scale our cardio efforts so that we are consistently making progress. I threw a lot at you, but I want to make sure that, before we go into strength training, we do not miss the most important thing about this section of the book. We want to make sure we are always moving. Our activity level is a MUST! We cannot have no movement at all. Our minimum is getting something done. This can be a 10 minute walk or 10 minutes of yoga at first, but the most important thing is that we are building good habits by doing something every single day. In the beginning, that is what matters. By doing this everyday, we are able to build positive momentum that creates a great base for us to build from. This is why I did not jump into high intensity in the beginning. Without having a foundation with the low intensity work, you'll end up like my trainer friend with a torn hamstring.

When it comes to sustainable weight loss, the greatest ability we can have is availability. Many athletes who are talented unfortunately have careers which don't last because they are always injured. This can happen to you and I as well if we are not remaining active and working to gradually get better day by day. It's said that excellence is a habit and it's built day by day. That is what I want you to walk away with after reading this section. We are building a habit that one day we will be excellent at performing. We are also ensuring that, when we get to the point where it is time to switch up our goals, we have the knowledge of high intensity cardio that we can use to make sure that our goals continue to trend upwards rather than stall out.

In the next section, we are going to be discussing strength training. Strength training is something that is very important if we are going to see results on our weight loss journey. When body transformation is something you want, strength training is an amazing tool to have in your toolbox. That is why we have it as part of our weekly checklist. It's not something you need to do everyday, but if you are going to see results and stay on the road towards the body goals you have, you do not want to skip or overlook some of the amazing benefits that it offers. We will also discuss how our cardio works hand and hand with our strength training, along with other things to be mindful of. It's not all about the work we do. It's also about how our bodies respond to the work and what we do BEFORE the work in terms of RECOVERY so we are set up to do our best work again.

I've been waiting to talk about this section for a while. As you know, I'm a powerlifter and always will be, so it's time to pick things up and put them down and push around some weights. Are you ready? Let's get to it.

Troubleshooting Cardio

- How will you track your cardio? For example, by steps, time, calories, or distance?

____

____

____

- We always like walking the best as a general recommendation. That said, based on your situation and experience, could you use other options detailed above? Which type of cardio is best for your body and your situation?

____

____

____

- List the modalities of cardio and related machines you have access to.

____

____

____

- List the exercises that you enjoy most, are easiest on your joints, and you are best able to recover from.

____

____

____

- How can you fit cardio into your schedule? Mornings? Evenings? Multiple short sessions or one longer workout? What will work for you? We are looking for any increase in activity level!

____

____

____

CHAPTER 6

STRENGTH TRAINING

For those who have been waiting for the weight lifting part of the book, we are here. For those who are not too crazy about weight lifting, you will be by the time we are done with this section. How can I be so sure? Because there are so many benefits to strength training that, when you see the wonders it will do to your body, you'll be sending me an email telling me that I should have talked about it sooner in the book.

To start, allow me to define strength training so we are both working from the same starting point. Strength training, which can also be referred to as resistance training by some, is a physical form of activity where you contract your muscles by use of an external source of resistance for the purpose of increasing muscular strength, muscular endurance, or both.

We will be diving into the different types of external sources of resistance we can use for the purpose of building strength, power, and endurance, but that is what it is in a nutshell.

As you expose your muscles to resistance, they will respond by developing in strength and size and what they are able to output. This is where one of the initial benefits of performing strength training comes in, at least when it is done correctly.

Progressive & Challenging

When performing strength training correctly, one of the goals is to get better from workout to workout. If you've ever heard from someone who regularly lifts weights, you'll always hear them tell you how they started lifting a certain weight and now they are able to lift a higher weight. For example, perhaps you started with 20 pounds on the bar and, after several weeks or months, you are able to double that weight and now lift 40 pounds on the bar. That is progress! The cool thing about strength training, when done well, is that it is progressive in nature. Have you ever wondered why those who do strength training are always seeing improvements with their bodies? This is a big reason for it.

One of the biggest things about having a progressive approach in your training is the fact you are still moving. You are doing something versus not doing something. You have something you are aiming for and aiming towards. Goals help move us. Without something to aim for or strive towards, it's easy to see why our results would come to a halt. But when we perform strength training, there is always another goal we can reach. We can lift heavier (muscular strength), we can lift a particular weight for more reps (muscular endurance), or we can both lift heavier weight and lift that heavier weight for more reps as our muscular strength and muscular endurance increases. This is one of the greatest benefits of strength training and why we have it as part of the checklist. You will be able to see sustainable results because the very framework of the program you are on is always moving forward and challenging you.

This also does wonders for not getting bored. When you are doing the same thing over and over again, it's easy to grow apathetic towards it and not want to do it anymore. That is where sustainability goes out the window and our results stop. Like we talked about going from low intensity to high intensity, the same thing can happen with strength training. You can always get better. Our potential and what is possible is not fixed. We can continue to grow and strive for greatness however we see fit. That's empowering and why I love this journey so much and why I'm so glad that you are on this journey with me. You have not seen the best version of you yet. The best of you is ahead of you.

Why Strength Training?

Another benefit of strength training is the fact that it helps us build muscle mass. The cool thing about building muscle mass is that muscle takes up less space in our bodies, so it allows us to weigh a certain amount but look completely different compared to other compositions that weight may represent. Here is what I mean by that. Sometimes when we are on this journey, we may see that the scale does not move and we interpret that as though we are failing. You do your daily weigh in and you do not see the scale move in the direction that you want. This has happened to you before, right? You're eating clean, you're getting in your 5,000 steps, at least, and still the scale is not moving. Well, when you are strength training, you can also add muscle mass which may make the scale not move, but it is much better to have 5 pounds of muscle instead of 5 pounds of fat. A pound is a pound, but what kind of pound it is makes a difference. Fat takes up more space than muscle. This means the more muscle mass we have the leaner we ultimately will look.

Muscle mass also helps us to have a higher metabolism which means we burn more calories throughout the day compared to someone who does not have as much. This is also why we have progress pictures and Inbody/Waist measurements as part of your weekly checklist. Too many times, people are actually making progress on their weight loss journey and are not aware of the progress they are making. Sometimes the scale does not tell us the complete story, but the progress pictures and the body fat or waist measurements tell us that we are actually moving in the right direction. This is what strength training can do for us. Are you now starting to see the benefits?

You do not have to be a "meathead" to take advantage of the benefits that come with strength training. Because you are tracking all the things you are doing, you have complete control on when to dial it up or dial it back, according to what your goals are. I know that, for those who love to powerlift, this section might come to us a lot easier than it may for someone who does not have a background in lifting. Nonetheless, do not be afraid of strength training.

Will strength training make me bulky?

This is a question I get a lot from people, women especially. The answer is that strength training won't make you look bulky as long as you know how to specifically manipulate your eating to ensure that it does not. In the next chapter, as we wrap up the book, we will be diving into the nutritional aspect of things, but note that there are many women that you can see on your social media channels who are not bulky and do strength training regularly. It is also worth noting that the bulky women you see are more on the extreme side in terms of what their nutrition is and what supplements they may or may not be taking to manipulate their hormones to look a particular way.

Types of Strength Training

Now, as far as the different types of strength training go, there are many different forms.

I won't go into too much detail in this book as there are many other books that speak of this extensively, but I do want you to be aware of the types at a foundational level so you are able to recognize them.

You can do strength training with your own body weight, for starters. You can do bodyweight squats, pushups, and other exercises like pull ups without having any external weight other than your own bodyweight. The key here is that it remains a challenging activity which can be adjusted (giving that progressive element).

Once you master your bodyweight, you can then use free weights such as barbells, dumbbells, and kettlebells. Other forms of resistance can be machines that have weights. These offer less stress on joints and, if you have balancing issues, the machine can remove that element to a degree. You can also use resistance bands and medicine balls to add resistance to your training. This where you might see stuff like medicine ball chest presses, ball slams for medicine balls, and curls, tricep pushdowns, and rows for resistance band work.

The cool thing about these options is you can use one of them or you can use all of them which gives us variety in our training and provides our bodies with different stimulants, so we can remain challenged and keep the progression training moving.

How Much And How Often

Now, how much strength training should we do and how often? For the purpose of fulfilling the requirement for our checklist, you will be strength training three times a week. That breakdown can be Monday, Wednesday, Friday or Tuesday, Thursday, Saturday. Again, whatever combination of three days works with your schedule is what is best. It's also important that we remember that we have to recover from the workouts we do as well, so you want to be mindful of that when you are training. You want to spread out the work. You do not want to squat on Monday, Tuesday, Wednesday, as that won't give your legs the opportunity to rest and recover so that you can give the proper effort the next time around.

You also want to factor in what your cardio activities are and what intensities you're using for your cardio as well. An important focus when it comes to scheduling strength training sessions and cardio sessions is simply when they are done. Sometimes you will have someone do strength training for their legs on Monday and then on Tuesday plan to do a high intensity cardio session. This may not be the best because your legs will be beat up from the Monday strength training session and you will not be able to perform at a high intensity level the following day. It's at this point you want to schedule a low intensity cardio training (which you have to do everyday anyway) the next day. If you want to schedule a high intensity cardio training day, it's probably best to just add it to your strength training session, especially if the focus is a leg day where you are squatting or doing deadlifts. Because the high intensity cardio is not a long session, you can easily tack on an additional 5-15 minutes at the end of your strength training workout and get the benefits of burning more calories, enjoy that "afterburn effect", and help your body continue to burn calories for 24-72 hours without running the risk of injuring yourself or not being able to recover fast enough, costing you that consistency which is so integral to this program.

You can also join our Facebook group, where we have sample routines available in the resources section, so you can ask any questions you have along the way about how to incorporate this. If you'd like more assistance or one-on-one guidance, our coaching programs are great to get that high level of attention and fully understand how to take your training and results to the next level. This is not necessary, but if that is something that you see would help you along in your journey, by all means, use it.

Now that we've covered the working out portion of the book, it's time for the one part every body transformation program or weight loss program covers: nutrition. We saved one of the best things for last in this one. We're almost to the end of the book and you've done an amazing job staying with us the entire way as we have learned the fundamental building blocks that will allow us to troubleshoot our own weight loss and fat loss journeys.

Troubleshooting Strength Training

- What kind of strength training is best for you to start with?

___

___

- List modalities, machines, and tools you have access to, whether they are included in a home gym or a separate facility. Do you have a coach? Do you need one?

___

___

- Are you working around any injuries or preexisting conditions? Are there any body parts or movements you want to strengthen specifically? Do you have any strength or performance goals?

___

___

- Based on these answers, what would your ideal workout look like?

___

___

- On what 3 days could you set aside some time for working out?

___

___

In case it helps you out, I'll quickly note some of the finer details of my personal workout schedule. Remember, your own will likely look different! I work out more days a week, and often more days in a row, than I recommend to those just getting started. You'll notice I utilize different schedules for different goals. That is an essential part of our approach!

When my goals tend towards powerlifting and strength
Sun: Squat and lower body focus
Tues: Bench and upper body focus
Thurs: Deadlift and lower body focus
Fri: Upper body accessory based day

When my goals tend towards towards body composition and bodybuilding
Sun: Shoulders and arms
Mon: Legs and abs
Tues: Back and biceps
Wed: Chest and triceps
Thurs: Legs and abs
Fri: Arms and back

Feel free to sketch out a schedule like this for yourself below!

CHAPTER 7

PROTEIN

I have a question for you.

What is muscle's favorite macronutrient?

Okay, so that's not the best health and fitness riddle, but if you answered protein, you're correct! Protein is the building block that allows us to take the work we did in the last chapter with strength training to the next level. In this chapter, we are going to cover macronutrients and, in particular, our protein intake.

As listed in our daily checklist, eating more protein is one of the daily activities we need to do in order to have sustainable weight and fat loss. Everything stated in the daily checklist is a factor that can typically be out of whack and need troubleshooting. Protein is a big one. I've found that many people simply do not get enough of it to support the work they do in the gym. If our muscles repair and recover from our work with strength training by utilizing the protein we take in, then it's important that we make sure we are consuming enough protein to support this process.

For the sake of this section, we are going to strongly emphasize protein more than anything. People usually don't seem to have a problem with eating more fats or eating more carbohydrates, so that is why you will not see us really talk much about those within this section on nutrition.

Two Ways To Consume Your Protein

When it comes to consuming more protein, there are really two ways you can go about it. The first way is from whole foods. This is where we want the majority of your protein to come from. By whole foods, I do not mean the store. I'm talking about foods like fish, chicken, beef, etc. The other way you can go about consuming more protein is from supplementation. Depending on your goals and how much you weigh, both may be needed, while for others maybe just one is needed. For someone like myself who is a big boy, I personally need to get 200 to 250 grams of protein and that can be hard to come by just from food sources alone. This is why I get protein powders to help. This is the purpose of supplements. It's to make it easier for you to give your body what it needs to achieve the goals that you want. My favorite protein comes from 1st Phorm, in particular their Phormula-1 protein powder. I specifically like this because of the variety in flavors that they have. I personally really love the Loop D fruit and the CTC (Cinnamon Toast Crunch) flavor. I link to all of this in the resources section so you can get some of my go-to resources for getting my protein.

Make It Easy

There are many great sources by which you can obtain quality protein easily. During the pandemic, there was a program called The Give Program. For those who are not familiar with this program they delivered a box of the best source of proteins: locally sourced chicken, fish, shrimp, salmon, beef, and steak. Then, they gave a portion of the proceeds to help support local fitness trainers and gyms who have been impacted financially by the Covid-19 Pandemic. They have suspended their operations as of now, as far as I am aware, but you may be able to find a similar program local to you. Currently, I use a lot of Piedmontese Certified beef and get locally sourced seafood from Fish Foodies on Long Island. They deliver to surrounding states as well. If you are not in these areas or cannot use these sources specifically, the concept of getting your protein delivered to you can be helpful to stay on track. It just may require a little research on your part.

I share this with you for the sake of convenience. By having resources like The Give Program, 1st Phorm supplements, Fish Foodies, and Certified Piedmontese, I'm able to subscribe and order from each of them and have one less thing to worry about. When it comes to being consistent and having sustainability, the less you do, the better odds you have of being able to stick to your goals and accomplish all the things that you do need to do. We want to keep it super simple. You'll hear me share more about this a little bit later on when we cover improving our eating habits.

Protein Frequency/Feedings

When it comes to getting your protein intake, you'll want to aim for 3 to 6 feedings per day, depending on how much protein you need for your body. For me, I settle right around 4ish most of the time because a typical feeding for me will have about 50 grams of protein and I typically consume, at minimum, 200 grams of protein. For you, if you need to hit 150 grams of protein, that might be five feedings of

30 grams each or four feedings of about 35-40 grams per feeding.

This is where protein shakes come in. I typically have 1-2 shakes a day to help me get my protein easily. This helps me make sure I get the amount of protein I need on a daily basis so that I'm able to check off "eat more protein" on my checklist. Speaking of, how much protein should you be eating?

How much protein should you be eating?

For most men I recommend a minimum of 200 grams of protein and for women 150 grams of protein. This equates to about 4-6 six ounces of protein when you are using food sources like chicken, steak, beef, cod, salmon, or other fishes and protein sources. If you're like some people I know and don't want to eat that much protein, that is where a supplement like 1st Phorm's protein powder can come in and help ensure that you get your protein. I do realize that the reality that someone can sit down and eat 5 times a day might be challenging, but protein shakes make it a lot easier for you to just grab and be on the go without missing your daily commitments.

Benefits of Protein

Now, I know I've been preaching about eating more protein and you're probably sick and tired of hearing me say it, but here is why I am so big on it for this program. Proteins have a higher thermic effect when compared to other foods to help maintain muscle mass. A higher thermic effect simply means that your body requires more calories to digest, breakdown, and absorb the nutrients from the food. This is very good for those of us who are looking to lose weight and get more lean.

Another benefit of upping your protein is that you will see an increase in your recovery. When I cranked up my protein to 300 grams per day (not recommended for most), my recovery was much better. Before you go crazy and look at me side-eyed about how much protein I was consuming, I was training six days a week with weights, so my body needed that amount of protein. If there is a macronutrient that we need, I would be biased to protein over the other ones. It helps you maintain muscle and your body works harder to burn it, so we get more calories burned from it.

Carbs and Fats

But John, what do you have to say about Carbs and Fats?

As far as carbs and fats go, my short answer is that you should pick the path that best suits you. What you cannot have, however, is a high carb AND high fat diet. That will lead to too many calories, which will lead to weight gain. That's like eating donuts, pizza, pasta, and pancakes. Anyone with an eating plan of that magnitude is not going to see any weight loss happen for them.

When it comes to getting really lean, I will say that I have leaned towards consuming protein that is more on the lower spectrum when it comes to fat. For example, when you go shopping you will see 93% lean or 96-97% lean beef. This is really not for you unless you are on some cutting phase and want to make sure that you are really lean or plan to be competing on some stage. I just want to make mention of it to you in the case that you do come across it.

For carbs, you'll have some folks who subscribe to the notion that one should consume them in moderation, while others go straight keto and focus on high fat. An entire book can be written on this, but then we would be overwhelmed and stuck in the mud of excess information. For the purposes of this book, just know that we strongly recommend not being on both a high carb and high fat diet at the same time. This will make it very difficult to maintain a caloric deficit which is needed to drop weight. This is where tracking your food from the checklist will come in handy in the event you need to troubleshoot your results or lack thereof.

Nutrition and Protein Troubleshooting

- On average, how many meals a day is sustainable for you? This is your meal frequency. For example, I eat 4-5 meals a day with protein, on average

____

____

- What timeframe is sustainable for your meals to occur within? This is your feeding window. For me, this is 6:30 AM - 3:30 PM, on average.

____

____

- With your average feeding window and meal frequency, what would an ideal day look like for you. For example, I may eat at 6:30 AM, 8:45 AM, 12 PM, and 3:30 PM.

Ideally, you want evenly spaced meals throughout the day to maximize the effect of the protein. 4-5 meals a day has been proven to provide increased benefit from 2-3 a day.

___

___

- How will you track and plan your food intake? For example, you could use a food journal, the MyFitnessPal app, or take photos. Are you measuring your food or just estimating?

___

___

- What would be your preferred energy source: carbs or fats? Write down which you tend to eat more. More fatty foods or sugary foods? Do you feel better having more carbs or more fats in your diet? In general, we recommend around 60% or more of your total carb intake to be pre- and post-workout for optimal energy use. Even if you are on a low fat diet, you don't want it to get too low and impact your hormones. For more exact recommendations, you will want to work with a coach or dietician.

___

___

CHAPTER 8

HYDRATION

Raise your hand if you've seen someone with a jug of water in the gym.

Raise your hands and feet if they have cute motivational sayings on the water bottles too.

The next part of our checklist is hydration! It's an important step in the process of being healthy. Water is so crucial that anytime you hear someone get sick, what does the doctor always recommend? Drink lots of water. You've heard that before, right? It's been said that water is the best multivitamin that we can take. There are so many benefits to the body when we are properly hydrated.

For starters, water helps to regulate our body temperature and helps our body flush out what needs to be flushed out. Water also helps with our metabolism. We talked about adding muscle mass to help with our metabolism, but water is also a big part of it. Our bodies are made up mostly of water. Yes, we have our bones, muscle, and fat, but, according to studies, water can make-up up to 60% of our bodies. If something comprises that much of our body, it must be important and we want to make sure that we do not withhold our bodies from getting what it needs to operate at its best.

Hunger v. Thirst

Did you know that many times when you feel that you are hungry, you are really thirsty? We often mistake hunger for thirst. If you are feeling hungry, it may not mean that you are. It might just mean that you are in need of some water or some electrolytes. We'll talk about electrolytes in a second, but I wanted to share this with you because water does help big time in helping fight off those "hunger" cravings. Really, your body may be craving some fluids. Enter water and electrolytes.

When it comes to troubleshooting our weight loss journey, this is an area which, like sleep, can easily be overlooked. If your recovery is lagging or if you are feeling sluggish in workouts, water can be a big reason why. Let's dive into how much water we should be drinking.

How Much Water Should You Be Drinking

For men, I like to recommend at least four liters of water, or about a gallon, and for smaller people and women, about three liters per day. If your activity level is higher, or if it's hotter out, you may need more.

I personally like to knock out at least a liter first thing in the morning. This is a great way to get started and get into the habit of getting your water. There are studies that also show that drinking water can raise your resting metabolism up a fraction. When you are looking to lose weight and lose fat, a higher metabolism is your friend, so definitely drink more water!

Now, I know what you are probably going to say. I try to drink water, but I cannot go to the bathroom all day. I strongly recommend pacing yourself into drinking more water. If you do not drink water regularly, it might be a bit much to drink a gallon a day, for the men. For women or those who may not weigh as much, maybe 3 liters of water is a bit much right out of the gate. With everything in this book, it is about the build up. We build towards a certain point. As you make it a habit you will find it a lot easier to do and your body will get used to it. Especially if you do everything else in the checklist, your body is going to need an increase in water.

Nighttime Bathroom Runs

The one caveat with the water is to make sure you want to cut it at a certain point so it's not too close to bed. I've found myself waking up frequently in the middle of the night when I drink my water too close to bed. This, of course, can impact our quality of sleep. This is why I like to front-load my water early in the day by having a liter of water first thing in the morning and also having another around the time that I am going to train.

Electrolytes

If you've ever seen athletes on the sidelines when they are tired, what do you see them grab often? That Gatorade bottle, right? What they are really after are electrolytes. The body is not able to function at a high capacity when it is lacking proper hydration. You are not able to get your muscles to contract as you need to when it's in need of hydration. When athletes are dehydrated, you will often see them have muscle cramps. That is why they are constantly drinking water or electrolytes. If athletes, whose jobs depend on them being peak performers, are doing this, we too can incorporate this as a daily practice of our own, so we are able to make sure we are at our best to crush our goals.

When it comes to getting my electrolytes, I really love LMNT powder (you can find our affiliate link to this in the resources section). The LMNT powder comes in raw powder form (no flavor) and flavored powders. Essentially, it provides magnesium, potassium, and sodium. When you workout, you sweat, and in your sweat you lose these nutrients. Accordingly, they need to be replaced so that your muscles can contract.

I personally like to do at least a gram or a thousand milligrams of sodium before I work out and maybe even during the workout. These LMNT powders have a thousand milligrams of sodium, 200 milligrams of potassium, and 60 milligrams of magnesium. This is a really good ratio. To put in perspective, other foods that are rich in potassium are things like potatoes and spinach. Instead of having to eat those foods, you can supplement your efforts by drinking water with the LMNT powder in it. This is helpful especially if you are on a low-carb diet as you lean out and you are limiting your consumption of potatoes. You can still get your much needed potassium without the additional calories.

Hydration Troubleshooting

- What is your average water intake per day?
- If you do not already reach the goal of 3-4 liters, what is a simple thing you can do to ensure you are properly hydrated? For example, I drink 4 one liter bottles of

water a day. That helps to break down and quantify my progress so I can stay on track.

- Do you experience any dizziness, cramping, or signs of dehydration during training? If so, you may need to add more salt to your food or otherwise replenish your electrolytes.

- How will you replenish your electrolytes? You can add more salt to your meals, eat potassium rich foods or vegetables, or use a supplement such as LMNT powder which contains sodium, potassium, and magnesium.

CHAPTER 9

MEAL PREPARATION

If you fail to plan, you plan to fail.

I'm sure you have heard of this quote before. There's another version of the sentiment that is coined as the 5 Ps, which stands for:

1. Proper
2. Planning
3. Prevents
4. Poor
5. Performance

When it comes to troubleshooting your weight loss or fat loss, planning your meals or meal prepping, as we often call it now, is key. Studies have shown that meal prepping is one of the top habits of successful dieters, if not the most important habit. This, along with weighing yourself regularly, are big factors when it comes to weight loss and/ or fat loss. That's why it's on our checklist!

Meal Prep Twice A Week

We have incorporated this truth into our plan of action because we know that it works. We want to be set up for success and meal prepping is one of the ways to do just that. For our case, we want to make sure that we are meal prepping twice a week.

It's a lot easier to hit your goals when you have already planned the actions to ensure that they happen. Meal prepping makes it a lot easier to track your food (which is on the daily checklist). Meal prepping also makes it a lot easier to eat more protein (which is on the daily checklist). For me, I like to prepare meals on Sundays and Wednesdays. So, for me, that is right before the week starts and right at the middle of the week. You might have a schedule that may not allow that to be as easy for you, but, whatever the two days are for you, you want to make sure that you are doing it, period.

Beat The Hunger

If you are planning your food on the fly, your results will fly away with it too. This will take a little adjusting to if you have not done it before, but it's worked wonders for me when it comes to getting consistent and sustainable results with my training and nutrition. I once heard that we don't make the best decision when we are hungry. This is why we need to meal prep. You'll never have a bad day at work and say, "I'll go eat salmon with some asparagus". You'll easily go for the pancakes and all the fatty foods. This is where meal prepping is your friend.

Shop Same Day Of The Week

To make meal prepping a little easier, I recommend that you shop on the same day of the week each week. The fewer things you have to think about, the easier it is to get it done again and again. For me, it might be Sunday mornings right before I do my first day of meal prepping. For you, that might be while the kids are at soccer practice on Friday afternoon at the end of a school week. The key here is you want to be consistent. You can also tap into programs like The Give Program, local companies like Fish Foodies, both of which I shared earlier, or you can shop at Whole Foods through Amazon, if that is an option available to you. Take advantage of whatever food shopping and delivery options are available to you to make this as easy as it can be.

Variety Add-Ons

Now if you're one of those people that likes to have a little bit more variety and feel that oft-repeated things get stale, something that I recommend is using several varieties of hot sauces or zero carb dry rubs. There's a company called Keto Rubs which is good if you want zero carb seasonings. I like to use Frank's RedHot Sauce and Frank's RedHot Seasoning. Frank also sells a ranch powder. You can get creative with it to make sure your eating is not boring.

I really like Cholula hot sauce as well when I want to add some variety to my ground beef or chicken. After eating so much of it, I can completely understand the need for a switch up or kick every now and then.

You can also do different things in terms of salt and pepper and seasonings. Especially if you're local to Long Island, we recommend checking out Dudes Gourmet for this. They have an amazing array of spice and seasoning blends which make good cooking easy! In our resources section, you will see where we get our food protein and nutrient-dense foods and how we keep our meals fresh and fun while still hitting our daily and weekly checklist. Before we conclude this section on nutrition, we'd like to share with you some tips and tricks that you can use to help improve your eating habits.

How to improve your eating habits

Up to this point, we have shared about macronutrients, such as protein and water, and their value towards helping you with your weight loss and fat loss. Then, we discussed meal prepping. With meal prepping, you can ensure that you have a fail-proof plan and that you keep things interesting with your foods by making minor tweaks like adding a sauce or seasoning here and there. Now, we want to share some tips on how to improve your eating habits. The keyword here is improve. This means taking what you do now and making it a little bit better.

Too many times when it comes to improving our eating habits, our new habits don't stick because of how they were formed in the first place. Remember how I shared earlier how sometimes we can go in one direction so much that we can turn a strength to a weakness? I see this happen quite often with eating, as well. We go from 0 to 100 real quick, forgetting that both getting a result and keeping that result should be the goal. It is no use to just drop weight only to gain all of it back and then some. This is why the steps laid out in this book are designed to take the form of sustainable, doable actions that we can grow into over time. The question I ask myself when it comes to hitting my goals is, "how long do I want this to be my result?" For most, they do not think about this question and so their results don't stay for long. After learning the approach presented in this book, you will not be susceptible to this. It is clear what it takes to have complete control over your own weight loss and fitness journey.

Troubleshooting Eating Habits

- What days can you prepare meals?

____

____

- When can you regularly shop? List your best options to shop locally. I like Aldi's and BJ's/Costco. List your best options for foods you can get delivered. I like Certified Piedmontese and Fish Foodies.

____

____

- Are there hot sauces or seasonings which are zero or low calorie which you can use to spice up your meals? We like Dudes Gourmet.

____

____

- What is your confidence with your cooking ability? Not one of your strengths? Check out the resources section for our video cooking tutorials.

Here's an additional tip to put into practice when you are cooking! Use cooking sprays instead of oils. It is possible you may be missing a lot of calories in your tracking because you are not counting cooking oils. We recommend avocado or coconut spray specifically, as their smoke point is higher than other sprays.

CHAPTER 10

START WITH WHY

When it comes to your eating habits, I always like to ask myself and anyone that I work with, "why do you want to do what you're doing?" There is a book by Simon Sinek that has sold millions of copies called "Start With Why" where he talks about how great things come to be and also how they last. He talked about the company Apple and how their sustainability as a top flight company started with asking "why". It's definitely worth the read if you're into stuff like that, but, for the sake of this book, I want you to pause for a moment and think about your "why". Honestly sit down and ask yourself why you want what you want and why you are doing what you are doing or going to do. Think of yourself as a kid when your parents or an adult would ask you to do something and you would say "why".

This is a great place to start because it helps us to know if our "why", first, makes sense, and also if it is a strong enough motive to keep us on track with our journey. Is it sustainable, that motivation and drive for whatever your reason is? For example, for me, doing a bodybuilding show was something I wanted to do, but before I could really dive into pursuing that goal, I needed to know why I was doing it. If I was doing it just to get likes on Instagram, I would not have gone through the challenge that I did to complete the eight steps on the daily checklist, plus the steps on the weekly checklist. I would not get a program like The Give Program so I could make sure I had all my protein available to me. That "why" simply is not strong enough.

You might be wondering, "John, where are the eating habits tips, or why are you saying this?" Here's why. When I've asked people "why" they do some things when it comes to their nutrition, the reasons they give me are EXACTLY the reasons why they are not able to get sustainable results. This might sound a bit extreme, but it happens. I've asked someone why they decided to go on a ketogenic diet and the response will be "because I saw someone on Instagram on my explore page with abs do it, so I said why don't I do it too". Or they'll say, "I cannot drink my water because I cannot find non-GMO alkaline lavender essential oil infused water like Bossfitchicklifter123 on Instagram, so when I find it then I will start drinking water and making sure I get hydrated". As silly as this may seem, the reality is that it's done far too often. What we do not take into account is the "why" behind the post you saw on social media. Is their "why" because they got paid $5000 to do a sponsored post? Is their "why" because they have something specific they are looking to improve with their own body transformation journey that is COMPLETELY different from yours? You do not want to copy and paste everything someone else is doing. I'd rather you make the changes you make specific to yourself because you are the only person that matters in this journey. You are the driver and you chose the destination. While something can work for one person, it does not mean that it will work for you. This is even true for the stuff I shared in this book. Some of it won't work for you and for others it will. Maybe you don't want Frank's Hot Sauce or maybe when you get your protein powder you may not like the CTC flavor from 1stPhorm, but you'll understand the principles about needing more protein and can customize it to your specific needs.

Remember to be specific and honor YOUR WHY, not the why of someone else on the gram.

Troubleshooting Your Why

- Once you know what your goal is, ask yourself "why" seven times. Imagine a young kid asking their parents "why" over and over. Do that to your goal and write below where you end up.

____

____

____

____

- Is your "why" sustainable? Is it really yours? Do you really want it?

____

____

____

____

- "Is the juice worth the squeeze?" If your answer to the first "why" is that you want a six-pack, what is the answer to your seventh "why"? Which will get you to your goal?

For my example, I set a goal to squat 800 lbs in 6 weight classes. It was a challenge, but my numbers weren't really what mattered to me most. My goal, at the core, was to show others and myself that you can be lean, healthy, and still be strong. I wanted to show people what was possible. I didn't have to go from 340 lbs to a bodybuilding stage. The show was cancelled 6 times and I had already dropped the weight, but my goal was to show the end result of what was possible.

____

____

____

____

CHAPTER 11

TIPS AND RECAP

Exercise Patience

The next biggest issue, and this is a really big one, is P-A-T-I-E-N-C-E. It's amazing how we can wait so long for some things but we are not as patient when it comes to our bodies. We might give something a try in our fitness journey and then, after just three days, throw everything we've done out the window because we did not drop from a size 14 to a size 6 in a week or conclude that we did not drop five inches in our waist, so the plan must suck. Give yourself some time. Remember, if you want fast, it won't last. Slow and steady ensures that your results stick.

I have to admit that exercising patience is not an easy thing to do. We all want to get to the goal yesterday. This expectation, however, is not realistic and only leaves us with a flawed perspective which sabotages the potential of what could be possible for us. This is why we have so many ways to track your progress in this book. We realize that the scale is limited to one perspective, so it is easy to hone in on that one factor and think that everything is falling apart. So, what do you do then? You relax, you work your plan, and then at the end of the week you look at your measurements, you look at your progress reports, and you allow those additional data points to tell you a more complete story of what is happening. But do not just do this and say everything is going to be perfect in a week. Progression is the goal, not perfection. We are striving, moving forward, and making steps to get better and better as time goes on. Going at this pace allows you to see what is happening, giving you the ability to make adjustments as needed, but also to not add on additional stress on your body which can actually hurt your long term success with your weight loss and fat loss journey. Start off with trying to lose a pound a week. You don't have to drop five pounds a week like so and so did. Do you know that if you just lost a pound a week that in a year you'd be 52 pounds lighter? Even if you lost only half a pound a week, that is 26 pounds lighter. Don't think that's a big deal? Next time you workout, go find a 25 pound dumbbell and hold it over your head for a couple of minutes. Now, imagine if you could drop that weight and never have to walk with it again. That's more than likely for you. I'm a living testimony that it can happen.

Be Data Driven

When it comes to improving your eating habits, let the data drive you, not fads on social media or your own impatience. Data is your best friend when it comes to troubleshooting your weight loss. That is why we want to track our foods and that's why we want to use MyFitnessPal to track our level of activity. It's a lot easier to tweak what is also being measured. And, again, not everyone has to do everything on the checklist, but if you do log all that data, you will not be shooting in the dark with certain factors when it comes to making the adjustments you need. The checklist itself is your tool to ensure that you are able to collect the right data to ensure your success. Let that be your guide.

Use The K.I.S.S. Principle

When sticking to improving your eating habits and being consistent with them, you want to follow the K.I.S.S. principle. Some break it down as Keep It Simple Stupid, but I like to say Keep It Super Simple instead. The easier something is, the more likely you'll be able to do it and do it over and over again. The bigger the list, the bigger the change, and the more resistance you will have with it.

Look at any area of your life and tell me, when was the last time you made a huge shift in anything? Did you want to do it? What was your motivation like? Did it seem attainable to you? When we have something that totally disrupts our life, we will have a hard time doing it. But when you are focusing on a thing or two here and there, that is a lot more manageable.

It's like a juggler who is juggling balls in the air. One ball in the air is super easy, two balls in the air is not hard, but not as easy as one. Eight balls in the air, though, is super hard. Imagine 20 balls in the air. You wouldn't even bother. That is why, when we talked about sleep previously in the book, we said not to try to address all 3 of the Ts at once. Focus on timing first, then, when you get a handle on that, go with temperature. Or, maybe timing is a challenge for you right now, so start with temperature and sleep in some shorts and a tank with your socks off, if that is easier. Even with our checklist, we kept it super simple by giving you only eight daily steps and keeping the other steps weekly. Still, it's insane to expect you to be able to do all eight right out the box.

Remember, we are troubleshooting, which means we are addressing areas that need improvement and tweaking things after we track and measure what's going on. The simple wins more than the complicated. In fact, I love the quote that says, "simplicity is the ultimate sophistication." It can and will pay dividends for you.

Are You Set Up To Fail or Succeed

Speaking of sophistication and simplicity, a big part of success is in the setup. What do I mean by setup? Let me ask you this as a scenario. If Person A had a kitchen full of cookies and cakes and Person B had a kitchen full of protein powder for shakes and fruits and healthy nut options like almonds or peanuts, which person do you think would find success with their weight loss journey? Person B, right?

Why is that? Because Person B is set up for success while Person A is set up to fail. This is where I'm going to exercise a bit of tough love here, but if Oreos are your Achilles heel, how do they continue to find their way into your house? Now, you might say, "John, I don't do the grocery shopping. My significant other buys them". That's cool, but I need you to tell your significant other that you got goals and that they need to stop buying those cookies, or at least to buy them and eat them outside the house because that is just setting you up to fail.

Many people, and I've done this too, will think that the best way to see if you are disciplined is to have the Oreos in the house and you say no to them. Many would call this self-denial discipline. That sounds good in theory, until you have a person at work that pisses you off and you come home and make a mad dash to the cabinet and finish the entire bag of Oreos. There's a way to avoid this altogether. Set yourself up for success by not having it in the house at all. For you, it might not be Oreos, but you get the point that if you are serious about getting your body how you want it to be, about taking hold of your health, and if you have a strong enough "why", then this is what you will do.

Use Timers!

Your phone can be one incredible accountability partner on this journey when you utilize the timers. We know that we need to get more water, but sometimes it's easy to forget that we haven't drank it. Even with the water bottles that have the times on them, we can easily forget to drink it or grab it, especially when we are really busy at work. This is where using timers come in. Water is not an option in this journey. We have to have it. There are too many benefits to making sure we are properly hydrated to not do it. You can even change the label on the timer or alarm clock on your phone so that you are able to know why it is going off. Maybe for 8 AM, it's "jumpstart your metabolism", then at 11 AM you label it as "you are thirsty, not hungry". Whatever you do, just use what you have to set yourself up for success.

When we do this what we do is make all the steps on our checklist as foolproof as possible. The people who are able to find success think in advance about where they are going to fall and put things in place to make sure that doesn't happen. Think of it as some form of insurance. We get car insurance just in case we get into an accident. Even if we don't get into one we are protected. Is your eating protected? Is your hydration protected? Is your health and fitness protected? Did you think of all the possible potholes in the journey and put things in place to plug them up? That is what foolproofing your eating habits and this overall journey looks like.

Recap

We've covered a lot here for you so I want to bring us to a close with important points to remember. We know that protein is our good friend in the macronutrient world and how it helps us to maintain muscle mass, burn more calories, and help with recovery. Hydration isn't a luxury item but a necessity for us when it comes to keeping our cravings at bay, as we can often mistake hunger for thirst. We learned that when we plan our meals we are more likely to succeed and how it's one of the top habits that successful dieters use over and over to have continued success. And, lastly, we talked about practical strategies and tips you can use to take your eating to the next level. We know that it's crucial that our eating is dialed in and these tips were easy and super simple to implement so that you can be well on your way to achieving your goals and KEEPING THEM!

Troubleshooting Tips and Recap

This is a long troubleshooting section, so answer some of these now, as you can, but this is also a good section to revisit and reflect on your progress going forward!

- How can you empower yourself to exercise patience with your progress?

____

____

___

___

- Make sure to set reasonable expectations for your progress (no more than 1 lb a week, roughly). If the scale is not moving through a two week period, be more process rather than results oriented. Look at your data, look at your checklists. Are you nailing down every aspect? What progress have you made? What can you do to “stay the course”?

___

___

___

___

- One of the most important things about tracking is to utilize your results and make adjustments based on the information you collect. If we can’t measure, we can’t act on that knowledge, but to utilize it, we have to act. How can you react to the data you are collecting and stay data driven?

___

___

___

___

- If you are not achieving the results you want, how are you collecting data? Do you have accurate, consistent tracking? If yes, what daily minimum are you furthest from? How can you productively shift focus?

____

____

____

____

- How can you keep things simple? What can you tackle first? What should you add in later?

____

____

____

____

- Are there any environmental factors you can address (people, places, activities, projects) which take a lot of your energies? Can you change them? If not, what strategies can you use to get around them?

  Here are some examples I came up with:
  1. Have snacks for your kids? Make it inconvenient for you to get them. Generally "add friction" to getting to unhealthy foods.
  2. Out on business and going out to eat? Can you look at menus ahead of time or have regular orders to help account for calories?
  3. Big work deadline coming up? Can you shift your schedule? Maybe get up/go to sleep earlier to hit

items before you start? If you can't keep up with everything, what can you prioritize for the time being?

- Can you think of any other strategies to set yourself up for success, whether your environment can be changed or not?

- Are you overly critical of yourself? Yes? Feel like you are in a rut in terms of progress?
  A good exercise is gratitude journaling in the morning. Write 2-3 things you are grateful for when you wake up. Before bed, write the best thing you accomplished during the day. Again, dwell on accomplishments and progress. Be conscious of positive self talk. Be mindful: would you speak to a friend or loved one how you address yourself? Frame things in a positive way!

- Do you celebrate your small successes or do you need something grand to get excited? Are you a glass half empty or half full? It's okay either way. The most important thing is to be conscious of your mindset. Take inventory of it and act accordingly. For example, are swinging for the fences or aiming for consistency? The singles and doubles guy gets on base more than the big home run hitter, even if they both score the same amount of runs. If you can't take more strikeouts in between your big successes, maybe you are someone who needs consistent small successes to progress. Maybe you're the other way around. Each approach can work, but you have to understand your own temperament and adjust your mindset accordingly

---

CONCLUSION

You've made it.

We are at the end of this book and at the beginning of you taking ownership of your weight loss journey. The purpose of this book was not to overwhelm you with information, but instead to outline practical, small, actionable things you can do to troubleshoot your own weight loss/fat loss transformation.

Because of what you read in this book ,you have an idea of all the elements that produce sustainable weight loss. Anyone can lose weight, but it's about being able to keep it off. That is the challenge for many. You now possess the knowledge, strategies, and tools to be able to manipulate your weight as you see fit. If you want to add muscle, you know how to track your calories, how much protein you need to consume, as well as what your physical activity needs to be both in regards to resistance training and cardio. If you want to lose weight, you know the benefit of tracking what you eat using the MyFitnessPal app, the value of getting your 5,000 steps, and how much recovery plays towards you achieving great success with your weight loss journey.

For many years, this has been a struggle for me to conquer, but being able to consistently keep 100 pounds off my heaviest weight, to be able to accomplish all my in the gym goals and out the gym goals because of this checklist, this systemized approach has been life changing and empowering for me. It will be the case for you as well. No longer do you have to run to try the next new diet (which I promise you there will always be another one). No longer do you have to throw everything you know in the trash and run to copy the latest fitness social media model who swears there is only ONE thing that can get you results.

So, here's what is next for you. You have the tools and the strategies to control your weight as you want, it's now time to put the checklist to work. The only way to make progress is to move in the direction of your goals. As we've stated in this book, a GPS is pointless without a destination. Where do you want to go? Where do you want to be? The steps to getting there you now have.

If you are in need of more assistance or need to get a jump-start towards meeting your goals, I'd be glad to help you. At the end of this book, you will see a way for us to work together if that is something you feel would help accelerate your progress. Again, this is not necessary, however coaching has helped me to ensure success in areas where I have not in the past or where a little extra support was needed. If that is something you too need, we do have coaching programs where we walk alongside you to ensure that you are doing all the things laid out in this program. As I've shared before, many have dropped 20-30 pounds using this exact system and I have lost over 100 pounds and kept it off. Let's get you there too and make you the next walking, talking billboard, the next success story that shows that sustainable, small, actionable steps done consistently are the key to weight loss that never gets lost and is easily maintained.

Thank you for taking the time to read this book. It means a lot to me. It was the idea of knowing that, perhaps, I can help even one person overcome the struggles that have troubled me for years and which motivated me to first apply this entire system to myself and to write a book dedicated to you. Please share your wins with me by sending me an email at gaglionestrength@gmail.com. I'd love to hear how you're progressing both daily and weekly.

The power is now in your hands, go conquer your fitness goals like never before. You have what it takes.

RESOURCES

First, here is our linktree which features many of our resources, conveniently presented.
https://linktr.ee/gaglionestrength
Next, please email us at gaglionestrength@gmail.com for a copy of any of the images of the checklists or charts in the book.

G-Team Recommended Resources:

Codes are valid as of time of publication.

Supplements to crush your workout and recover better!
Free Shipping on 1stPhorm Supplements
https://1stphorm.com/?a_aid=gaglione

Stay on top of your electrolytes and hydration with LMNT!
LMNT Electrolyte Powder Referral Link (pre + intra workout)
http://elementallabs.refr.cc/johngaglione

Our buddies at Fish Foodies offer excellent, locally sourced seafood, shipped to you!
15% off your first order of Fish Foodies LI Local Sourced Seafood
Use code "GaglioneHealth" at Checkout
https://www.fishfoodies.com/

Get delicious, lean protein from Piedmontese
25% OFF Certified Piedmontese use Code "COACH" at check out
http://www.piedmontese.com/

Body Fat testing is a great metric to aid your progress!
Local Body Fat Testing: Use Code "GAGLIONE" for 50% Off
https://gettankedli.wpcomstaging.com/

Coaching with Gaglione Strength

Visit our website for information and events.
www.gaglionestrength.com

Sign up for a consultation here!
https://gaglionestrengthconsults.as.me/schedule.php

Check out these resources for more educational content, tutorials, and more!

Youtube:
https://www.youtube.com/c/GaglioneStrength/videos

Powerlifting for the People Podcast:
https://gaglionestrength.libsyn.com/podcast

Instagram:
https://www.instagram.com/gaglionestrength/

Facebook:
https://www.facebook.com/gaglionestrength/

ABOUT THE AUTHOR

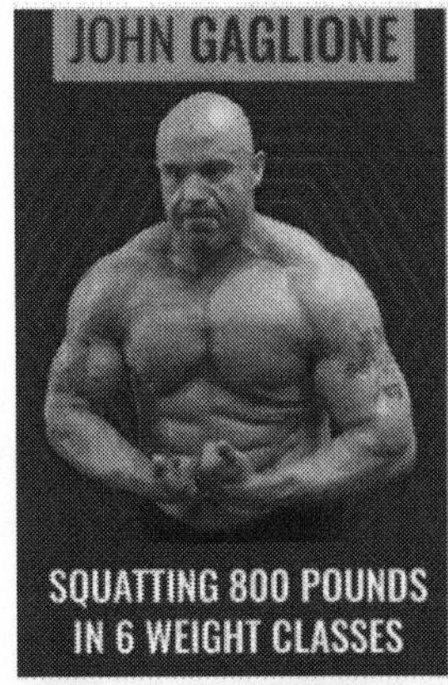

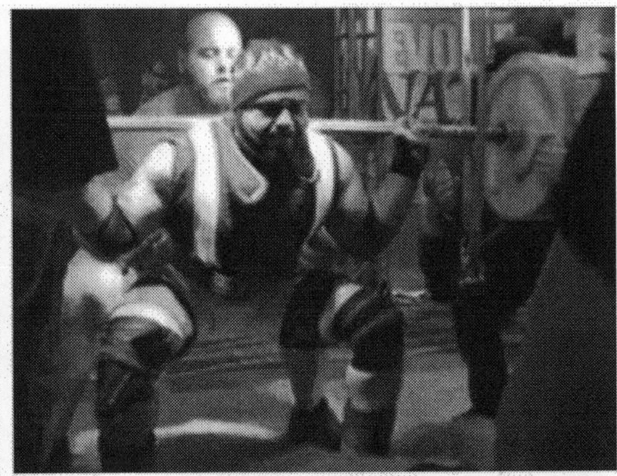

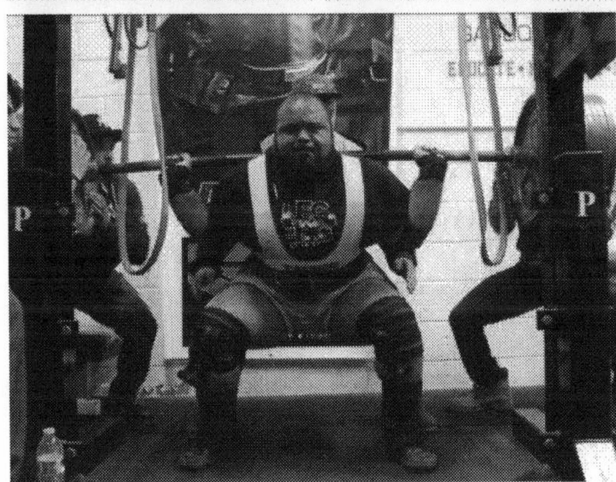

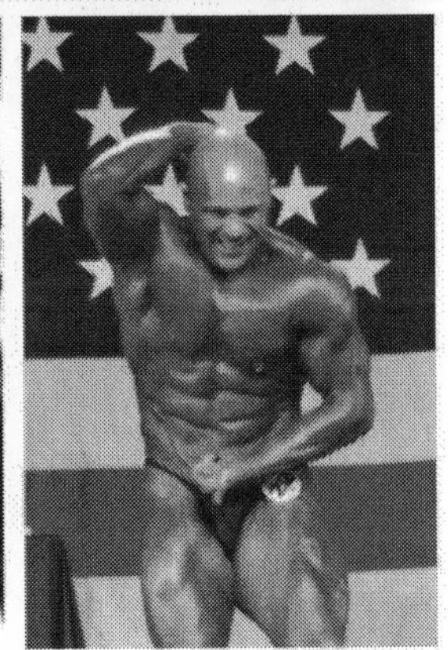

JOHN GAGLIONE

is a strength coach out of Long Island. John trains people from all walks of life at his facility in Farmingdale, NY. He specializes in improving maximal strength for athletes and "average Joes" alike and coaches the Gaglione Strength powerlifting team. Since the start of his coaching career, John and his team have trained at least 89 nationally ranked lifters.

He has written strength and conditioning articles for major online publications, such as Men's Health, Elite Fitness Systems, Testosterone Nation, One Result, and is a featured strength & conditioning author for the Long Island Wrestling Association. He has been a featured speaker for exercise science programs at several schools, including SUNY Cortland and Hofstra University

An experienced strength athlete himself, John has a lot of "under the bar" experience and has competed in the sport of powerlifting for over a decade. He has best competition lifts of a 900 squat, a 575 bench, and a 660 deadlift. Coach Gaglione is one of the only men in history to squat 800 lbs or more in 6 different weight classes. Recently, he has competed in an amatuer bodybuilding contest.

Made in the USA
Middletown, DE
11 August 2021